Facing impending death: Experiences of patients and their nurses

Gina Copp
PhD, MN, DipN(Lond), RCNT, RGN

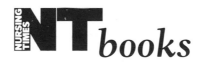

Acknowledgements

My grateful thanks go to all those who helped with this book, especially, of course, the patients and their nurses who are its core.

For Lucy

All names in case studies have been changed.

First published 1999 by Nursing Times Books
Emap Healthcare Ltd, part of Emap Business Communications
Greater London House
Hampstead Road
London NW1 7EJ

Text © 1999 Gina Copp

Printed and bound in Great Britain by Drogher Press, Christchurch, Dorset.

British Library cataloguing in Publication Data
A catalogue record for this book is available from the British Library.

ISBN: 1 902499 15 8

Contents

Preface: Origins   v

I   RESEARCH INTO DEATH AND DYING:
        A REVIEW OF THE LITERATURE   1

1   Death, dying and nursing   3

2   Current theories of death and dying   36

3   Review of methods and tools used in studies
        on death and dying in health care settings   50

II   EXPLORING THE EXPERIENCES OF
        PATIENTS AND THEIR NURSES   55

4   Analysing accounts of patients' experiences
        and those of their nurses   57

5   Case summaries   70

6   'Taking each day as it comes'   109

7   'Past my sell-by date'   134

8   'I don't know how to die'   156

III   DYING AND NURSING   195

9   Conclusion: implications for nurse practice,
        theory development and future research   197

IV   APPENDICES   213

     1: Focus and design of the study   215

     II: General approach and research strategies
        in the study   223

V   POSTSCRIPT, REFERENCES AND INDEX   237

     Postscript   239

     References   244

     Index   267

Preface: Origins

My early nursing experience exposed me to numerous dying patients and the issue of confronting death. Most of the deaths I witnessed were in acute hospitals, were generally unexpected and involved patients who were often too ill to regain consciousness and therefore prepare for their deaths. On reflection, the feelings I experienced as I nursed those patients were not dissimilar to those experienced by other nurses (Field, 1984, 1987; 1989; James, 1986; Smith, 1992; Kiger, 1994). There were occasions of dread, tempered with humour, fear, sadness, sorrow and horror, particularly when mutilated bodies of children and adults arrived at the A&E department. Most of the time the immediacy of the situations demanded that I carry on, incorporating and accommodating dying and death as aspects of life's misfortunes.

Some years ago, before embarking on the study that forms the core of this book (part II, pp 55 194), I made a significant change of career by moving into palliative care. This term describes the total care offered by a team of doctors, nurses, therapists, social workers and volunteers to patients whose disease is no longer responsive to curative treatment (World Health Organization, 1990). The goal is to achieve the best possible quality of life for patients and their families by taking into account the physical, psychological, social and spiritual aspects of care. This approach has its origins in the early works of the hospice movement (Saunders, 1970; Saunders, Summers and Teller, 1981, Taylor, 1983), particularly the pioneering work of pain relief, symptom control and humane care for the dying. These have profoundly influenced, and are widely acknowledged as providing, the foundations for current palliative care services (Abel, 1986; Seale, 1989). Today, hospice care is based on an approach that affirms life, while at the same time acknowledging that dying is a normal process.

Since their inception hospices, and the translation of hospice philosophy into other health care settings, have generated considerable interest (James, 1986; Seale, 1989), as well as remaining topical (Douglas, 1992; James and Field, 1992; Clark, 1993a; Field, 1994). This is exemplified by the range of work on both the historical and future developments of hospices and the impact of hospice philosophy across different health care settings (Wilkes, 1980; Seale, 1989; Standing Medical Advisory and Standing Nursing and Midwifery Advisory Committee Joint Working Party on Palliative Care, 1992). For instance, the growth of the hospice movement has been argued as a counter response to the euthanasia movement (James, 1986). The success of hospice care may be attributed to the emphasis of the patient as a total individual, to the inclusion of their family in decisions about care and to using both professional and lay skills in providing care and hope in the presence of death. Although this tradition is, to some extent, an alternative to mainstream care, Clark (1993a) has pointed out that hospices do not exist in isolation from mainstream health care. Indeed, the introduction of an internal market (Department of Health, 1989) posed new challenges for hospices, including greater external scrutiny, working in a competitive environment and having less independence and autonomy.

In my case, the change from acute to palliative care occurred more by accident than design, motivated mostly by personal curiosity and a desire to deepen my understanding of the nature of nursing care of the dying. At the time, hospice nursing represented to me the pinnacle of quality nursing. For instance, in contrast to acute care settings the hospice ethos of teamwork, commitment and open discussion of patients' prognoses and the fostering of nurse-patient relationships (Field and James, 1993) was an attractive option. I was curious to find out more about the nature of this care and to learn from the experience. In particular, I was hoping to learn more about caring for patients who were aware of their impending death, in direct contrast to those patients in my previous nursing experience who often did not have the opportunity to know, or talk about, or prepare for their death. To gain this experience I started work in a local NHS hospice and began my grounding in palliative care as a novice nurse by working on the ward. The following provides an account of a situation in which I was struck by the expression of a dying patient on the ward while working on a late shift one evening.

Mary, a patient in her 60s, had been in the ward for a week. She had been unwell and was admitted for pain relief and symptom control. During the evening she suddenly ran out of her room shouting loudly: 'I am going to die, I am going to die.' My initial reaction was a mixture of fear and bewilderment. It was a situation I had not come across before. However, I moved quickly over to Mary and, putting my arm around her shoulders, we sat down, Mary talked and I listened. Gradually, she appeared less anxious. I walked her back to her bed and settled her with a cup of hot chocolate, remaining with her until she began to fall asleep. Mary died the next day.

This and other related experiences stayed with me, adding to my curiosity about the process of dying and death and the responses of nurses. These observations raised fundamental questions about how people express their experiences of dying. Mary's differed from that of most patients on the ward. Was her ability to express it so vocally related to feeling safe to do so, or was it a consequence of mounting fear that had not been expressed until that moment? I was unsure of the answer, yet felt I needed a deeper understanding in order to respond appropriately to Mary's call for help.

Reflecting further on experiences of a number of dying patients like Mary led me to ask the following questions:

- In what ways do different people express their experiences of dying?

- What is the relationship between patients' expressions of dying and the responses of nurses? For instance, reflecting back on my experience with Mary, it was clear that fear and uncertainty had been aroused within me, yet my response was diametrically opposite to my inner feelings of wanting to run away.

- How did I overcome this fear?

- What made me respond in the way I did?

Little has been published in UK nursing literature on the experiences of people who were aware of their impending deaths or the experiences of nurses who care for them. There have been no studies to date that have attempted both to capture the depth of experiences of dying patients and to gain insight into responses of nurses who care for them. This is surprising, as most patients are willing to talk about their experiences. Moreover, experienced palliative care nurses possess a wealth of practical knowledge regarding their responses to dying patients. Most of the time, this knowledge is used by experienced nurses to illuminate points or to validate common expressions of dying. However, much of this practice knowledge remains implicit (Duke and Copp, 1991) and, unless opportunities arise for overt discussion; it disappears, being accommodated into individual nurses' repertoires with little or limited contribution to the general body of knowledge in nursing.

It seemed to me, therefore, that a potentially valuable approach would be to document cases of patients' experiences of their dying and of nurses' responses to caring for them. The strength of this approach is that it provides information about practice in a practice context. The study of individual cases of patients and the responses of their nurses would provide data that could be used to examine current theories of death and dying. Thus, it was from a position of nursing practice, stimulated by human curiosity about experiences of real people, that this work on experiences of dying originated and evolved.

THEORETICAL BASIS OF THE STUDY

In order to gain insight into patients' and nurses' experiences simultaneously, the theoretical approach used draws on a symbolic-interactionist perspective (for review, see Denzin, 1992) within an interpretive interactionist framework (Denzin, 1989a). The basis of this approach is that all human beings interact and the basis for that interaction is dependent upon language and actions, which are in themselves symbolic, simply because meanings of experiences are often shared and conveyed within interactions (Blumer, 1969). These meanings are not just conveyed but are also shaped by the self-reflections that people bring to situations. For instance, human conduct is not governed solely by 'stimulus-response' relationships (Mead, 1964). It involves a greater degree of flexibility, including the capacity for planning ahead and revising future conduct by reflecting on the outcomes of individual actions and interactions with others. Mead (1964) attributes this to the self-awareness of human beings. This aspect of a person's make-up gives rise to an individual with the capacity to be both subject and object at the same time, in any environment.

In a recent review on the historical development of symbolic interactionism, Denzin (1992) draws on a host of seminal and current works (James, 1890; Dewey, 1896; Mead, 1934; Strauss, 1959; Blumer, 1962; Stone, 1962; Garfinkel, 1967; Goffman, 1983) to classify and examine the contributions of the different schools and generations of symbolic interactionists, from the turn of this century to the present. In the context of Denzin's review, it is clear that the strength of symbolic interactionism lies in its pragmatism and its commitment to view knowledge as being close to the workings of the world. However, as a theoretical perspective it is more complex and comes in a variety of forms and approaches: dramaturgical, political, discursive, negotiated order and so on. In an attempt to synthesise some of these perspectives, Denzin (1989b, p.7) coined the term 'interpretive interactionism' to combine traditional symbolic interactionist thoughts with other interpretive approaches. This is exemplified in Denzin's (1992) recent attempts to integrate some of the key features of traditional symbolic interactionist thoughts with other interpretive approaches by presenting a synthesis of these approaches within an interpretive interactionist framework. Denzin (1992, p.26) writes:

'The interactional order (Goffman, 1983) is shaped by negotiated, situated, temporal, biographical, and taken-for-granted processes (Garfinkel, 1967). The central object to be negotiated in interaction is personal identity or the self-meanings of the person (Stone, 1962; Strauss, 1959; Couch et al, 1986). These identities, which are personal (names), circumstantial (age, gender), and social or structural (professor, student) range across the modes of self-identification just described. The meanings of identity lie in the interaction process and emerge and shift as persons establish and negotiate the task at hand (Couch et al, 1986). The situations of interaction may be routinised, ritualised or highly problematic. Within them consequential experience occurs. Epiphanic experiences rupture routines and lives and provoke radical redefinitions of the self. In moments of epiphany, people redefine themselves. Epiphanies are connected to turning-point experiences (Strauss, 1959). Interpretive interactionists study epiphanic experiences. The interactionist locates epiphanies in those interactional situations in which personal troubles become public issues (Denzin, 1989). In this way, the personal is connected to the structural, through biographical and interactional experiences.'

In my thesis, the epiphanic (Denzin, 1989b) or turning-point experiences (Strauss, 1959) described by Denzin (1992) above are defined as those that are confronted by people during the period of time between the crisis of knowledge of death and the point of death. This period of time has been described by Pattison (1977) as the 'living-dying interval', comprising phases of acute crisis — for instance, knowledge of impending death, chronic living-dying, and eventually a terminal phase. I would argue that the interactional sequences that give meaning to this period of experience as people face impending death, and their construction of those experiences in relation to other people and vice versa, are central to how we locate and redefine ourselves during problems.

In conducting the study my own experiences with the participants also contributed to my, and their, overall experiences. This is in keeping with the interpretive interactionist perspective (Denzin, 1992). That is, the researcher's experiences contribute and are an integral part of the overall data. This is inevitable. In order to understand someone's experiences, there is clearly a need to establish a relationship with them. Whenever possible, therefore, I have tried to include and describe the nature and depth of my relationship with the participants.

Patients' deaths evoked sadness and grief in me. These feelings, combined with the need to 'resurrect and relive' their experiences in order to interpret and write about them, were very difficult at times. Although at one level the process and outcomes were sad, the experience I gained from pursuing this work was, in many ways, positive and enriching.

1: Research into death and dying: a review of the literature

1. Death, dying and nursing

THE NATURE OF DEATH AND DYING

'All the recent literature in our society about death and dying — our pathographies, our scholarship, the popularizations of Elizabeth Kübler-Ross's ideas on the stages of dying and grief, recent Broadway plays and television specials on death — reflect our cultural search for viable models of "how" to die. We have no art of dying appropriate to the problems created by our advanced medical technology — no generally accepted model that would serve both to contain and to express the intense feelings that this most painful experience calls forth. Today, as Larry Churchill points out, "each (person) is as unique an individual in dying as in living. Nobody dies by the book."'

(Hawkins, 1991, p.302)

Death and dying have been subjects of intense study throughout the centuries from artistic, philosophical, religious and medical perspectives. In Western culture, this is immediately evident when examining contemporary and ancient works of literature, music and art. This reached a peak in medieval and renaissance cultures at a time when traditional Christian beliefs and rituals for death were jointly expressed in various art forms, thus codifying a set of beliefs, convictions, attitudes and practices regarding death (Kastenbaum and Kastenbaum, 1989; Hawkins, 1991). Recently, some authors have argued that, far from being a taboo subject, the public interest in death and dying has increased, as exemplified by the deluge of deaths being portrayed in plays, art, books and the media (Duclow, 1981; Walter, 1991; Walter, 1994).

Duclow proposed that society may be moving towards a contemporary equivalent of the traditional artistic view. Walter argued that the subject of death is currently undergoing a revival in western society. However, it is in a form that is individualistic rather than collective, because the traditional shared norms of how to die and mourn have now disappeared. The question of whether new beliefs have been created is contentious, however. For example, Hawkins (1991) argued that the considerable number of narratives concentrating on the search for a good death served as counter-evidence — they indicate the lack of a single art of dying.

The study of death and dying extends beyond art forms to linguistic analysis. For instance, the terms 'death' and 'dying' have also been subjected to scrutiny, particularly in attempts to define and distinguish them. There appears to be a general consensus that death should be viewed as an event and dying as a 'process'. A closer analysis shows the complexity of these two concepts. The definition of death has become increasingly problematic, as medical science and technology continue to make advances. Death is not usually an instantaneous process and, in the initial stages, may even be reversible if the right technology and skills are available. The latter has led to considerable attempts during the second half of this century to establish medical criteria for death (Backer, Hannon and Russell, 1982; Veatch, 1989). Accompanying these developments have been moral and ethical debates on whether such approaches prolong life, or the process of dying.

The concept of dying, on the other hand, indicates a process. According to Smart (1968a), this is in part due to our use of language. For example, 'to die' uses an active verb, and implicit in its use is the notion that somehow the act arises from the individual, as opposed to the case of being killed. Further, dying is viewed within the context of dying of a condition, as opposed to the person being the cause of the dying. This is normally accompanied by an awareness of the process of dying. Yet to say that a person is dying of something does not mean he or she will die of that condition. There are the possibilities of either sudden death intervening (such as by accident) or the person being rescued from the predicament of facing death. Thus Smart (1968a) says: 'It is not surprising that the ordinary-language concept of dying should be increasingly hard to apply in hospital situations, where the resources for dramatic interference in the normal sequences of disease are so vastly multiplied.'

Definitions of death and dying have not, however, decreased our fear of death. Morbid fears of burial before death are common in ancient literature (Mant, 1968; Alexander, 1980). In a more academic way, death and individuals' fear of it have contributed to philosophical and metaphysical expositions on concepts such as anxiety, existence of the after-life and the meaning of life (Frankl, 1962; Toynbee, Mant, Smart et al, 1968; Hanfling, 1992). Philosophical movements, such as epicureanism, stoicism, Christianity and, more recently, existentialism, have made profound impacts on the search for an understanding of the origins and nature of death and the meaning of existence. But in general it would appear that most authors share a common view — that death is a paradox. For instance, Collinson (1992; p.153) asserts that, according to Heideggerian view, it is only through the realisation of one's death that a person can begin to confront 'the absurdity of finding oneself inhabiting a life that was preceded by nothing and will be succeeded by nothing'. This paradox, once understood, makes clear the role of personal responsibility for existence and being. This is because being surrounded by nothingness renders everything meaningless unless the person is willing to make something of the present life.

Unlike Heidegger (1926), Sartre (1958), cited by Littlewood (1992), views death as unlikely to give meaning to life in itself. Sartre considers death 'in terms of the loss of the self in particular, rather than in terms of life's meaning in general' (Littlewood, 1992. p.74).

According to Sartre, the 'self' involves two aspects: being for others and being for self, and death involves the loss of being for self. Following death, the second aspect of the self, 'being for others' remains, as memories. Consequently, contrary to current bereavement literature, which tends to view 'anticipatory grief' from the perspective of those about to be bereaved (Parkes and Weiss, 1983; Rando, 1988) it is not unusual or surprising to find that the person facing death also experiences anticipatory grief, including the grief of 'being no more'.

Aldrich (1963) postulated that the type of grief experienced by the dying in response to anticipated losses (including all human relationships through death) is not too different from the notion of anticipatory grief experienced by relatives of the dying. Using Venn diagrams to illustrate interpersonal relationships, Aldrich (1963) showed that proportionally, when compared to the loss that will be experienced by the dying person's friend or relative, theoretically, the dying person's losses would be equal to the sum of the losses of all those friends and relatives. Aldrich argued that, all things being equal, a person who has the capacity for forming many meaningful ties and relationships with others is more likely to experience greater grief. However, Aldrich's proposal is clearly a demonstration only of how grief may arise for some people. Human relationships are complex and, as Rando (1988) pointed out, the experience of grief arises not only from anticipated or future losses but also losses that have already occurred and those that are currently happening.

Although it has been widely acknowledged that dying people experience grief as they face progressive loss of control, there is little empirical work on the grief of dying people in comparison to the work on the bereaved. Consequently, the understanding of the loss of being for self is still limited (Copp, 1996).

Existentialist thoughts have often been perceived as arising from despair in the face of absurdity. Most societies have traditionally sought comfort in the belief that there is more to human existence than life on earth. This is exemplified by beliefs in a spiritual world, reincarnation, or an eternal life after death. The latter forms the heart of traditional Christian conviction and is attractive, particularly when compared to the rather limited measures available to preserve life, which, according to Hinton (1984), merely serve to provide a brief pause. However, the belief in the after-life has increasingly become a contentious one (Toynbee, 1968; Smart, 1968b) and has been challenged by the growth of a scientific attitude and a secular society.

Writing about the philosophical concepts of death, Smart (1968a), suggested that our attitudes to birth and death are asymmetrical. When contemplating death, the thought of future non-existence seems more disturbing than past non-existence. Basing his argument on an existentialist perspective, Smart argued that this is, in part, a consequence of our inclination to view death as a mockery of life's achievements — because ultimately, the existence of death suggests that we are nothing, even though there was a time when we were nothing before birth. Yet we seldom think of birth or conception as mocking us. This may be because we exist in a structure of human activities that is open rather than closed, directed to an end, with a sense of anticipation, such as a future generation or future variations on a host of other activities. Human concerns are, therefore, mainly future-orientated, and the notion of this future is used on occasions to justify the present.

Contemplations on death also raise a broader debate about the point and value of human activities and existence (Smart, 1968b). This is particularly evident when one considers that moral and ethical issues, such as the sanctity and preservation of life, are paradoxically bound within the context of death and individuals' fear of it. This notion of fear had been further expounded by Choron's (1964) philosophical analysis of *Mortality and the Modern Man*. Choron used material from history and literature to demonstrate several death fears: fear of what comes after death, fear of the event of dying and fear of ceasing to be. Fear of the dead is also experienced by some, although Choron considered this as separate from the other three types of fear. Kastenbaum and Aisenberg (1972) pointed out that all three types may be experienced, in any combination.

From a philosophical viewpoint, there is clearly some relevance in reflecting on the meaning of death and dying, and of life and living. Equally, it is unsurprising that entertaining thoughts of death and dying may evoke feelings of apprehension. This apprehension, or dread, has been observed to contain both fear and anxiety (Schulz, 1979), although, as Hinton (1984) argues, much of it is normal and has biological value. For instance, fear originates from genetically determined instincts and from individual experience and is a vital element of human constitution. Without the fear of death, lives would be risked unnecessarily.

Drawing on the works of psychoanalysts, Schulz (1979) tried to distinguish between fear and anxiety. Schulz asserts that fear is experienced in response to specific environmental events or objects, such as pain. In contrast, anxiety is a negative emotional state that lacks a specific object. For instance, thoughts of death and dying may arouse amorphous and unspecified anxieties about the many unknowns connected with death. Moreover, it is this anxiety of 'non-being' that makes thinking about death unsettling and incomprehensible for some. Much of the thinking behind this is based on Freud's (1957) observations relating to death. For instance, in *Zeitgemässes über Krieg und Tod (Thoughts for the Times of War and Death)*, Freud (1957, p.289), wrote: 'It is indeed impossible to imagine our own death; and whenever we attempt to do so we can perceive that we are, in fact, still present as spectators. Hence the psychoanalytic school could venture on the assertion that at the bottom no one believes in his own death, or to put the same thing in another way, that in the unconscious everyone of us is convinced of his own immortality.'

Within this Freudian view, any imagination of our own death is virtually impossible, as we must continue to exist and can only act as spectators. This has been suggested, in part, as an explanation of why thoughts of death are anxiety-provoking and difficult to deal with. Weisman (1972, p.13), however, argues that it is not the 'result of consciousness being unable to conceive its negation' but rather that death is continually denied and perceived because 'it is other people who die, to the extent that, when man grieves, it is because he has lost someone significant to him, not because their death foreshadows his own.' According to Weisman, it is this fusion of death and denial in man's original make-up that constitutes the primary paradox of man. The very existence of death provides two distinct functions: it is both a destructive and creative force. As Schulz (1979) sums up, it is the experience of fear and anxiety about death that serve to motivate much of human behaviour, either directly or indirectly, contributing both to human neurosis and psychosis, as well as many good works and creations (Becker, 1973; Meyer, 1975; McCarthy, 1980; Rainey, 1988).

Summary

I have focused on elucidating the more esoteric elements of the nature, meaning and purpose of death (and, in so doing, aspects of the meaning of life) that have fascinated philosophers for centuries. Consequently, it is not surprising that philosophical discourse on this subject has continued with frequent renewed analyses, debates and viewpoints on classic works, as well as more contemporary thoughts on the meaning of life and death (for a review, see Hanfling, 1992). However, more pragmatically, much of the fear of death may be argued as tangible and real, arising out of observations and/or real life experiences of death and the process of dying (Twycross and Lichter, 1993). For instance, for some people the processes of dying are either experienced or observed as painful, frightening, humiliating and inconvenient, involving interruption of life's goals and separation from loved ones, and are tempered with regrets, both for self and others. Seldom are dying and death seen positively, except as a release from suffering or in instances of martyrdom. Moreover, as Smart (1968a) highlighted, the person who is aware that they are dying is also aware of the way in which they are dying. This makes the experience of living with dying a difficult and frightening one for most people. The rest of this chapter will explore some of physical, psychological and social influences of death and dying.

THE EXPERIENCE OF DYING

'...Suddenly he felt the old familiar, dull, gnawing pain, the same obstinate, steady serious pain. In his mouth there was the same familiar loathsome taste. His heart sank, his brain felt dazed... "Yes, once there was life and now it is drifting away, drifting away, and I can't stop it... Yes, why deceive myself? Isn't it obvious to everyone but me that I am dying and that it's only a matter of weeks, days...it may happen this very moment." A cold chill came over him, his breathing ceased, and he heard only the throbbing of his heart.

"I shall be no more, then what will there be? There will be nothing. Then where shall I be when I am no more? Can this be dying? No, I will not have it!" He jumped up and tried to light a candle, fumbled about with trembling hands, dropped candle and candlestick on the floor, and fell back upon the pillow.

'That Caius — man in the abstract — was mortal, was perfectly correct, but he was not Caius, nor man in the abstract: he had always been a creature, quite, quite different from all others... Caius was certainly mortal, and it was right for him to die; but for me, little Vanya, Ivan Ilyich, with all my thoughts and emotions, it's a different matter altogether. It cannot be that I ought to die, that would be too terrible.'

(Tolstoy 1960, pp.135-137)

In *The Death of Ivan Ilyich and Other Stories,* Tolstoy graphically portrayed the expressions and thoughts that ran through Ivan's mind when he realised he might be dying. As the story of Ivan Ilyich highlighted, a person who is aware of the way in which they are dying is in a situation that directly contrasts with, and yet incorporates, the Freudian viewpoint of consciousness not being able to view its own end. The prospect of imminent death involves the person in 'living with the process of dying', and watching the impact of this on their own body and life.

Physical influences and processes

At the turn of the century, from his analysis of 500 dying patients' records, Osler (1906, p.36) found '...90 patients suffered bodily pain or distress of one sort or another, 11 showed mental apprehension, two positive terror, one expressed physical exaltation, one bitter remorse. The great majority gave no signs one way or the other; like their birth, their death was a sleep and a forgetting.' Since then the physical processes of fatal illness, and their consequent impact on a person's well-being, have been extensively described (Charles-Edwards, 1983; Hinton, 1984; Lindley-Davis, 1991; Newbury, 1991, Seeland, 1991; Nuland,1994). Most of the information on fatal illnesses has tended to focus on chronic diseases, such as strokes and advanced cancer, where time is available to collect data and observe both the care and treatment provided. Lingering deaths, particularly from malignant diseases, have generally been associated with pain, suffering and discomfort. The concept of 'total pain' in the dying (which demonstrates the multiple facets of physical, psychological, social and spiritual elements), first introduced by Saunders (1985), has become widely accepted and established as the basis for treating and understanding the impact of pain on individuals (World Health Organization, 1990, p.21). While most people would prefer a quick and painless death rather than a slow, lingering one, most deaths from disease are not quick and involve time spent in hospitals (Hinton, 1984). People may experience gradual physical deterioration, loss of bodily functions and varying degrees of pain and discomfort.

The process of physical deterioration varies and depends to a large extent on the nature of the disease and the circumstances of care and treatment. For some, they may appear subtle, with minimal changes for much of the time, whereas for others, physical deterioration may be more obvious. Most people, particularly those with advanced cancer, experience some or all of the following symptoms: pain, incontinence, nausea and vomiting, breathlessness, noisy breathing, inability to swallow and feelings of weakness and malaise (Lichter and Hunt, 1990; Lindley-Davis, 1991; Back, 1992).

Much of the literature on the processes involved in dying from advanced cancer has focused on overt signs of deterioration that become increasingly obvious as the terminal phase approaches. Physical indicators include the person being profoundly weak, essentially bedbound, drowsy for extended periods, disorientated for time, severely limited in attention span, lacking interest in food and fluid, and experiencing difficulty with swallowing (Twycross and Lichter, 1993). Studies have also concentrated on symptoms, level of consciousness and the relationship between symptoms, biochemical indices and prediction of life expectancy (Witzel, 1975; Cerny et al, 1987; Foster and Lynn, 1989; Saunders, 1989; Lichter and Hunt, 1990; Ventafridda et al, 1990; Rosenthal et al, 1993). Symptoms such as pain, dyspnoea, urinary dysfunction, incontinence, restlessness, agitation and noisy breathing appear common as death approaches (Lichter and Hunt, 1990; Ventafridda et al, 1990). Although previous studies on levels of consciousness before death are difficult to compare because of the variations in measures used, it has nevertheless been reported that 6-30% of patients remain conscious until within 15 minutes of death (Twycross and Lichter, 1993).

In contrast, studies investigating the relationship between symptoms (and life expectancy) and prediction of life expectancy have yielded mixed results (Cerny et al, 1987; Reuben et al, 1988; Rosenthal et al, 1993; Addington-Hall et al, 1990). Rosenthal et al collected data on 148 patients from two hospices over a 15-month period in order to determine whether there is a relationship between 19 clinical and laboratory parameters and the duration of survival. The investigation showed that four factors were significant. Patients were unlikely to survive more than a week if they required admission at first referral, showed elevated serum bilirubin, hypotension and poor scores as measured by the Eastern Co-operative Oncology Group (ECOG) performance status tool. In contrast, patients who showed none of these factors survived between one and three months.

Performance status does appear to be an important predictor of life expectancy (Cerny et al, 1987; Reuben et al, 1988; Rosenthal et al, 1993), but few other measures have been confirmed as significant predictors. For instance, hyponatraemia, confusion, tumour type and weight loss have all been associated with shortened survival in hospice patients (DeWys et al, 1980; Reuben et al, 1988; Forster and Lynn, 1989), but were unconfirmed in Rosenthal et al's (1993) study. One problem may be a lack of uniform use of indices between studies.

The literature on physical aspects of cancer deaths has tended to focus on symptomology and causes of impending death, rather than on the physiological processes that lead to death. These remain largely uninvestigated and have been open to various speculations. For instance, although drugs have contributed to symptoms such as confusion, restlessness, and twitching (seen in the days preceding death), it has been argued, alternatively, that these symptoms, together with others, such as pain, dyspnoea, nausea and vomiting, form a much wider picture of cumulative multi-organ failure, which is largely multi-factorial (Lichter and Hunt, 1990; Martinson and Neelon, 1994).

It seems logical that death eventually occurs as a result of failure of normal physiological functioning of cardiovascular and respiratory systems. For example, as Hinton (1984), Nuland (1994), and Martinson and Neelon (1994) pointed out, diseases such as cancers, vascular disorders and strokes either interrupt or damage blood supply leading to eventual death when the damage is extensive. Acute infections may kill either by damaging body structures directly or through the spread of toxic products that damage vital centres such as the brain stem. Some malignancies secrete hormone-like substances (such as cachectin) that have direct effects on nutrition, immunity and other vital metabolic functions in the body (Nuland, 1994). Nonetheless, towards the end of life a number of vital processes often decline simultaneously. The view that the flow of vital fluids is crucial to life and that stopping the movement of liquids and gases at a cellular and organismic level constitutes death have long served as distinguishing features for advocates of the traditional concept of death.

Psychological influences and processes

The psychological processes of death are invariably linked with the perception of death and dying and the emotions that may be evoked. The nature of death and dying is paradoxically linked to individuals' fear of them, giving rise to anxiety and dread. It is not uncommon to find that a life-threatening condition, such as a diagnosis of an incurable disease, may precipitate a psychological crisis by arousing anxiety. The word anxiety arises from the Latin *anxius*, meaning to press tight or to strangle (Lewis, 1967) and carries meanings associated with emotional unease, often accompanied by physiological bodily changes — for instance, clammy extremities, dizziness, dry mouth, nausea, vomiting, and a fast pulse (Lader and Marks, 1971).

The early literature on the psychological processes of death and dying were predominantly psychoanalytical approaches. However, in recent years researchers with a psychodynamic orientation have extended this work to clinical situations using methods independent of psychoanalysis. Moreover, eclectic approaches adopted by researchers on this subject have also contributed to a broader understanding of the psychological elements of dying, in particular, death anxiety and its relationship with factors such as age, sex, religion and physical health.

Drawing on Cullberg's (1970; 1971) works, Qvarnstrom (1978, p.20) asserts that 'anxiety and defences against anxiety form central concepts in psychodynamic theories'. Thus, when anxiety is evoked, such as in death and dying, defences are activated simultaneously in the attempt to control that anxiety. This intricate interplay of anxiety and defences is important as a function for survival. Some of the defence mechanisms observed include denial, repression, projection, reaction formation, regression and rationalisation (Qvarnstrom, 1978). Of these, denial appears to be the most frequently used, suggesting the inherent anxiety that consistently recurs when someone has to confront mortality.

The term 'ego function' has been identified by various investigators as central to our understanding of responses to death and dying (Weisman, 1972; Pattison, 1977; Qvarnstrom, 1978). Pattison pointed out that the term 'ego' refers to a set of mental operations, the 'ego set', within which lie several functions, such as a sense of the self and personal identity. The ego may therefore be conceived as the control centre of the self, 'interposited between the unconscious drives, images, fantasies, and impulses, and the external world of reality' (Pattison, 1977, p.309). It has often been postulated within psychoanalytical theory that, when the ego experiences problems in resolving conflicts between the internal unconscious self and the world of reality, a variety of ego defences are used to deal with these threats.

Although ego defences, and their links with Freudian concepts of neurosis, have been seen as mainly pathological, some authors caution against directly applying and interpreting psychological responses in dying people (Dumont and Foss, 1972; Weisman, 1972; 1984; Pattison, 1977). For instance, not all ego defences are pathological and under stress most people (including those who are dying), resort to the use of what are called 'immature' coping mechanisms, such as acting out, projection and denial through fantasy. The central issue, as Pattison (1977) emphasised, is not about using defence mechanisms, but whether the mechanisms that are being used are adaptive, or helpful.

The use of denial as a defence mechanism has generated considerable debate (Weisman, 1972; Pattison, 1977; Taylor, 1983; Rando, 1984; Hughes, 1986; Rainey, 1988; Russell, 1993; Smith, 1993). These debates have arisen as a direct response to the popular, but negative, interpretation of denial by some health care professionals (Rainey, 1988; Russell, 1993; Smith, 1993). This was compounded further by Kübler-Ross's (1969) labelling of denial as an individual's initial response to terminal illness. Denial became perceived as negative, the least mature response to a terminal illness. In contrast, acceptance was viewed positively.

Clinical studies have shown that dying people can use denial as a sole defence, or they may exhibit elements of partial denial at different times (Kübler-Ross, 1969; Weisman, 1972; Pattison, 1977; Qvarnstrom, 1978). In his authoritative work, *On Dying and Denying,* Weisman (1972) provided data to elucidate theoretical expositions on the concept of denial. For instance, he showed that denial consists of an 'act' and a 'fact', both the act of denying and the fact of denial depending on personal interaction 'to define what, how and when denying takes place' (Weisman, 1972, p.61).

The most significant contribution of Weisman's work is in providing a fundamental understanding of how these processes work by distinguishing between degrees of denial that Weisman called first-, second- and third-order denial. First-order denial (of facts) occurs when there is an unequivocal refusal to accept the primary facts of illness or disease — for instance, when marked discrepancy occurs between a person's report of his condition and what is observed by another. Second-order denial (of implications) refers to people who accept the primary facts of their illness and diagnosis but continue to deny the implications of the long-term outcome of their illness. This is often observed in the form of reluctance to comment about the future and use of rationalisations to explain exacerbations or setbacks. Third-order denial (of extinction) refers to people who have already accepted the facts of their illness and are facing imminent death but on occasions resist acknowledging the finite nature of their situation.

From his case material, Weisman (1972, p.65) observed that an 'area of uncertain certainty' exists between open acknowledgement of death and its utter repudiation. In other words, people fluctuate between denial and acceptance. Weisman called this phenomenon 'middle knowledge'. Middle knowledge tends to occur at critical transition points, such as when someone begins the descent towards death or experiences setbacks. More recently, reviews on the use of denial in cancer patients have drawn attention to a number of studies that have shown their use of frank and partial denials (Hughes, 1986; Barraclough, 1994). Evidence from the studies suggest that people use different forms of denial by delaying seeking consultations despite suspicious symptoms, in coping with knowledge of diagnosis and in the terminal stages of dying. Hughes (1986) further highlighted that partial denial is used by most cancer patients who, although complying with various treatments for their cancer, often do not openly acknowledge their diagnosis.

Clearly, denial is frequently used as a means of coping. By providing a safety net, albeit a temporary one, it appears that denial serves to preserve self-esteem, maintain control and prevent disintegration and chaos. Moreover, acts of denial exist only from inferred observations of conduct or speech. This implies that any suggestion of denial must be considered in the light of interpersonal relationships. It has been suggested that denial operates not merely to avoid threat but also to preserve existing relationships (Weisman and Hackett, 1967; Weisman, 1972; Rainey, 1988; Smith, 1993).

The question of whether the same defence mechanisms are used throughout the human life cycle has interested a number of investigators. Pattison (1977) identified the types as well as frequencies of typical 'ego-coping' mechanisms used throughout the life cycle (Table 1). There appears to be a general trend from 'primitive' to 'mature' ego-coping mechanisms along a developmental sequence.

Table 1. Typical ego-coping mechanisms of the dying throughout the life cycle (Pattison, 1977)

Ego-coping mechanisms	Early childhood	School age child	Adolescence	Young adult	Middle age	Aged
Level 1 – Primitive						
Delusions	+	+				
Perceptual hallucination	+	+				
Depersonalisation	+	+				
Reality-distorting denial	I	I				
Level 2 – Immature						
Projection	++	+++	+		+	
Denial through fantasy	++	+	+			
Hypochondriasis		++	++	++	++	+++
Passive-aggressiveness		+++	++	+++	++	++
Acting-out behaviour		+++	++	+++	++	
Level 3 - Neurotic						
Intellectualisation		+++	+	+++	+	
Displacement		++	++	+		
Reaction formation		++	+++	+		
Emotional dissociation		+++	+	+	+	
Level 4 – Mature						
Altruism		+		+	++	
Humour			+	+	+	+
Suppression			++	+++	+++	+
Anticipatory thought			+++	+++	+++	+++
Sublimation			+	+	++	+++

+ = occasional use   ++ = moderate use   +++ = frequent use

Reproduced with the kind permission of Simon & Schuster from *The Experience of Dying* by E. Mansell Pattison. © 1977 by Prentice Hall Inc.

Alongside the work on psychodynamic responses of dying people there have been a considerable number of investigations on death anxiety. This research prevailed in the 1960s and 1970s, when interest in anxiety and coping mechanisms were equally popular with other behavioural psychological theories (Lazarus, 1966; Speilberger, 1966; Lader, 1969). Factors such as sex, age, religion and ill health have been found to relate to death anxiety in a number of studies (for review, see Schulz, 1978).

Studies using Templer's (1970) Death Anxiety Scale (DAS) showed that women feared death more than men (Templer, Ruff and Franks, 1971; Iamarino, 1975). However, when subcomponents of death anxiety are analysed, other investigators found that men have more fears of the effects of their deaths on dependants (Diggory and Rothman, 1961), and violent deaths (Lowry, 1965). Moreover, male death anxiety tends to be cognitive and female death anxiety more emotional (Degner, 1974; Krieger, Epsting and Leitner, 1974). These outcomes depend on whether an affective scale, such as Templer's (1970) Death Anxiety Scale, or a cognitive scale, such as the Krieger, Epsting and Leitner's (1974) Threat Index, is used (Schulz, 1978).

Studies on the relationship between death anxiety and age have been inconclusive, although there is some pertinent data relating to children's developmental phases to their perception of deaths. Nagy (1959) interviewed 378 boys and girls, aged between three and 10 years, and showed that, between the ages of three and five, death is perceived as a temporary departure, or sleep, between the ages of five and nine it is seen as final and from the age of nine onwards as final and also inevitable. On the other hand, attempts to investigate whether there is a relationship between death anxiety and age in young, middle-aged and elderly adults have been inconclusive, although elderly people tend to have lower death anxiety than young and middle-aged adults (Lester and Templer, 1993). There are probably confounding variables in studies of this type, however, including the presence of unconscious denial, (Schultz, 1978) and individuals' concept of death (Lester and Templer, 1993). Moreover, within families, positive correlations have been found between the death anxiety of adolescents and their parents and between husbands and wives, with especially high correlations being observed for same sex dyads (Lester and Templer, 1993).

The relationship between religion and death anxiety has been investigated by a number of researchers (Hinton, 1963; Lester, 1967; Lester, 1972; Feifel and Branscombe, 1973; Feifel, 1974). Early studies were inconclusive, perhaps because of conceptualisations of religiosity (Schulz, 1978). Subsequent studies have been careful to distinguish between indicators of extrinsic religiosity (frequency of church attendance, for example) and fundamental values. These studies have shown that the degree of religiosity, as measured by church attendance and belief, is unrelated to death anxiety in the general population (Templer, 1970; Feifel, 1974), but when there is fundamental religious involvement, death anxiety is lower (Templer, 1972; Shearer, 1973). Personality, temperament and life experience affect the way individuals live out their religious lives, so extrinsic measurements of religiosity remain contentious. In recent years attempts have been made to adopt a more eclectic approach by incorporating measurements of state and trait anxieties, as well as religious and existentialist dimensions, within the concept of spiritual well-being (Kaczorowski, 1989; Peterson and Greil, 1990). On balance, it appears that deeply religious and non-religious people tend to have lower death anxiety than those with weakly held beliefs (Hinton, 1963; Templer, 1993).

Investigations of death anxiety have also explored relationships between death anxiety and ill health. The 'two-factor' theory postulates that death anxiety is related to general psychological health and to specific experiences surrounding death (Templer, 1976). Limited evidence from an earlier investigation (Templer, 1970) showed that people who were less physically healthy tended to report higher death anxiety than healthy people, although subsequent studies did not support these earlier findings (for a review, see Schulz, 1979). Patients with psychiatric illness consistently showed more death anxiety than those without, and scales of death anxiety also continue to show positive correlations between anxiety, depression and existential uneasiness (Lester and Templer, 1993).

Although experimental studies on the influence of factors such as sex, age, religion and ill health on death anxiety have been popular in previous investigations, they remain inconclusive, despite considerable attempts to define concepts and develop measurement tools. Such studies are also confounded by the fact that death anxiety may fluctuate, depending on circumstances and the level of support provided. It was not my intention to study specific factors of age, sex and religion on their own, nor discount the value they may play within the patients' relationships. The age and sex of people was therefore taken into account when asking patients to participate. Age and sex provide specific indications of an individual's location and role responsibilities within the family life cycle. Individual beliefs (religious and non-religious), on the other hand, are taken into account during the course of the study, recognising that beliefs are dynamic and may change during the process of dying (see Chapter 7). These factors are seen as important in terms of how people construct meaning during dying and death.

Social influences and processes

Although the physical and psychological aspects of death and dying embody what are essentially private experiences, the social phenomena of death and dying arise directly out of a collection of these experiences. Demographic factors, such as birth and death rates, assert considerable influence on the beliefs and practices of people in relation to death and dying (Pine, 1980; Field, 1994). The experience of death and dying is therefore rooted in the culture of societies, contributing to varied beliefs and practices. The social organisations of death and dying are often seen as important and symbolic of how everyday living is conducted among members of a particular society (Charmaz, 1980; Clark, 1990; Clark, 1993b). According to Pine (1980), social organisations can be seen to involve at least three levels of interactions. At its most basic level, they concern the face-to-face contact between individuals. The second level is often related to relationships at a group level; that is, between and within individuals of different groups. The third level reflects the overall patterns and characteristics of group existence, thus creating a sense of social order at a societal level. Many of the social influences and processes of dying may be located at all three levels.

Deaths have been viewed as phenomena that cause disruptions within the social order of society. Giddens (1991) coined the term 'ontological security' to refer to individuals' sense of order and continuity in relation to events that govern their everyday lives. According to Giddens, ontological security depends on us being able to find meanings in our lives. However, this security is constantly under threat from chaos or disorder. Therefore, society attempts to contain this threat by 'bracketing out' those questions regarding social frameworks that govern human existence. An event such as death disrupts social order and poses a threat to individuals' ontological security. Consequently, we often find rules and rituals being performed to mark the passage of death (Van Gennep, 1960; Blauner, 1966; Littlewood, 1993) as part of a social response to contain the 'chaos' produced by death. Funeral rites are not only for the disposal of the dead but also for the benefit of the living and bereaved, by reaffirming social values, acting as a means to separate the dead from the living and providing an occasion for groups to assemble, in order to mourn and grieve.

Recently, such views have been challenged. In a paper focusing on the relationship between self-identity and the structuring of death in contemporary social life, Mellor and Shilling (1993) argued that the increased identification of the self with the body and a 'shrinkage in the scope of the sacred' have tended to privatise people's experience of death. Thus, the organisation and experience of death have become increasingly privatised and there is a trend towards 'keeping death at bay'. This is marked by a reluctance to come into contact with the dying, an orientation towards a youth culture, parents' reluctance to acquaint children with facts about death and the increasing medicalisation of death. Moreover, when death occurs, the event continues as a relatively private and hidden affair, marked by few rituals but accompanied by an increased uneasiness about the boundaries between the corporeal bodies of the living and the dead.

Even at funeral services, Mellor and Schilling pointed out that instead of dealing with death and dying as meaningful events of everyday life, it has become a collective trend to shy away from mortality. Death occurs in private but is absent from public domains. Walter (1994) criticised this view, pointing out the considerable body of public discussion on the subject, for example, in medicine, in health service planning, in life insurance predictions and in the media. According to Walter there is a mismatch between the private and public realms of the social management of modern death. Walter also argues that the shift towards a post-modern western individualistic culture has led to the belief that people should choose the way they wish to die and be mourned. Consequently, death and dying are increasingly being shaped by individuals (often at the invitation of doctors and nurses), rather than by the dogmas of religion or the institution of medicine. This post-modern 'revival of death' ensures that the individual sets their own dying agenda. So, as public rituals surrounding death continue to decrease, and death has 'died' as a social event, at the same time it is also being 'revived' in an individualised form. Walter concludes by saying 'dying and grief are increasingly being done my way'.

Unlike in previous centuries, most deaths and dying now occur in institutions. While it was common for deaths to occur at home in the early part of this century, by the end of the 1980s, 71% of the population in the UK was dying in institutions, compared with 23% at home (Field and James, 1993). This institutionalisation of dying has remained topical and has been the focus of much discussion, particularly in the area of institutionalisation of western societies (for a review, see Sweeting and Gilhooly, 1992).

Several explanations have been proposed for this trend (Blauner, 1966; Elias, 1985; Field, 1989; Kellehear, 1993). The fragmentation of extended families and the focus on individualisation have increasingly been seen as promoting a culture of self-reliance, with the emphasis of not becoming financial and personal burdens on family members. When balanced against the costs of care at home, the offer of 24-hour medical and nursing attention in institutions appears attractive, particularly for those who are chronically ill. Thus, care often shifts from homes to institutions.

The increase in life expectancy has also meant that death and dying have become primarily the experience of the old. In his classic work, Blauner (1966) outlined the increasing impact this has on the social processes of death and dying in the USA. Similarly, in the UK, Field (1989, p.5) highlighted that, as a result of the decrease in mortality rates in the young, there has been a significant increase in the number of people who survive beyond working age. Recent statistics (Central Statistical Office, 1992) showed that in 1991 there were 2.1 million people over the age of 80. Those aged 60 and over have risen by a third since 1961, to 12 million people, and this figure is projected to rise by over half to reach more than 18 million in 2031 (CSO, 1995).

Not only are younger people infrequently exposed to death and dying but, as Blauner argues, the dead are also missed less today than in previous centuries. This is because, previously, death often occurred in the prime of life, leaving behind social, economic and psychological gaps to be filled. By contrast, the deaths of the elderly members of contemporary society do not leave the same noticeable gaps. Combined with increased management of death by hospitals and funeral organisations and a decrease in shared values, meanings and rituals, modern death and dying have become phenomena that are, to a large extent lonely, unfamiliar, to be feared, denied and avoided (Gorer, 1965; Becker, 1973; Elias, 1985).

Several investigators have examined the social processes that have encouraged the trend towards death and dying in institutions (Glaser and Strauss, 1965; Gorer, 1965; Blauner, 1966; Sudnow, 1967; Illich, 1977; Aries, 1983; James, 1986; Field, 1987; 1989). Aries (1983) traced the changing attitudes of western societies towards death from a historical viewpoint. Control of the dying process and the place of death have changed significantly between contemporary society and those in previous centuries (Littlewood, 1992). Previously, dying and death were at the heart of communities and controlled by the individual, families and communities. Today, the sick and the dying are cared for in institutions and dying and death are primarily controlled by the medical profession (Field, 1994; Walter, 1994). This has been suggested to have occurred as a consequence of a pervasive but misguided belief in society that death could be conquered with the progress of medical science (Illich, 1976).

It has also become increasingly likely that the dying person's last days may be spent with strangers, separated from families and friends (Sudnow, 1967; Corr, 1993). In his study of death in two hospitals, Sudnow (1967) also showed that hospital staff employed different ways of dealing with the dying, particularly in attempts of resuscitation. The higher the perception of a person's social worth, the greater the efforts were made at resuscitating them. Of particular significance is Sudnow's conception of the term 'social death'. In order to distinguish social death from clinical and biological deaths, Sudnow tried to define these three terms. So, clinical death occurs following death signs at physical examination and biological death happens when cellular activities cease. Social death, in contrast, 'is marked by that point at which the patient is treated essentially as a corpse, though perhaps still "clinically and biologically" alive'. The socially relevant attributes of the person therefore 'begin permanently to cease to be operative as conditions for treating him', and he is 'essentially regarded as already dead' (Sudnow, 1967, p.74). According to Mulkay and Ernst (1991), when social death occurs a person may be involved in numerous social death sequences. These sequences could be conceived as interactional processes, operating over long periods of time. Moreover, these people may be perceived as socially dead by some but socially alive for others.

This rather bleak portrayal of dying in contemporary society has been further illuminated in recent discussions (see Kellehear, 1993) that are critical of institutional treatment of the dying, in particular the disclosure of bad news and the dominance of impersonal hospital routines over personalised care. Glaser and Strauss's (1965) classic study *Awareness of Dying* showed how patients in institutions are often unaware that they are dying, the news being withheld by staff so that patients have to resort to picking up cues and attempting to confirm their suspicion. Staff also adopt a variety of strategies to circumvent disclosure of bad prognosis (for a detailed discussion see Chapter 2). Armstrong (1987, p.653) postulated that doctors may have used the notion of 'secret' as a strategy to withhold bad prognosis. This, Armstrong pointed out, helped to justify the view that the 'truth about death cannot be told' in order to maintain the patient's hope. Armstrong said that 'the secret could in mysterious ways pass between doctor and patient without speech'. Silence is therefore seen as a conspiracy, yet desired by both the doctor and the patient in overcoming embarrassment, and in not confirming the patient's worst fears.

Schou (1993) conducted a longitudinal study of 33 cancer patients receiving radiotherapy in an out-patient department. By analysing their narratives, Schou highlighted that the 'awareness context' of these patients appeared ambiguous and concluded that 'treatment calendars' are often used by doctors as the means of protecting the 'secret of dying'. Clearly, disclosure of cancer is complex. As James (1993) illustrated in three reports of her interviews with patients, disclosure involves emotions. During disclosure, there are different levels of involvement with feelings associated with cancer and from competing forms of status and knowledge.

Citing Blauner (1966), Kellehear (1993, p.14) pointed out that hospitals have become mass reduction systems for 'reducing pain, death, sickness, independence, and individuality to sanitised, compliant and pyjamaed patients'. Hospitals, Kellehear argues further, are 'largely responsible for the depersonalisation of modern death'. Although most people would agree that hospitals tend to be impersonal, there has been little consideration of possible alternatives for the dying. What is needed is direct comparison, substantiated by evidence, of individual cultural contexts of dying in the present and previous centuries.

In contemporary society the range, effects and perceptions of care provided for the dying tend to vary, as shown in Hinton's (1979) study, which compared places and policies for terminal care.

More recently, there has been evidence to suggest that conditions for dying in UK hospitals may have improved (Seale, 1989). This has been demonstrated by comparative studies between St Christopher's Hospice and local London hospitals, using a number of outcome measures, including pain relief (Parkes and Parkes, 1984). Also, given a philosophy of individualised patient care, together with a supportive, open and non-hierarchical style of relationship between staff, care of the dying can be humane and personalised. This was shown by Field (1987; 1989) who explored nurses' experiences of caring for the dying.

The social organisation of death and dying operates at its most basic level, in face-to-face interactions and relationships between people. This is particularly true between members of families, in terms of how affairs of death and dying are conducted, and re-enacted, from one generation to the next. Much of the research in this area has been conducted in the field of family therapy and relies on the assumption that families operate on the basis of rules, patterns of relationships and beliefs. One of the more popular approaches in this field is the use of systems theory (Bennum,

1988; Burnham and Harris, 1988), where members of the family are seen in terms of sub-systems. Each person depends on the other for appropriate functioning and adaptation. A family system may either be closed or open, with the latter being preferable if adapting to change is to be successful. Such changes would include major events like births, deaths, illnesses, unemployment and family members leaving home.

Underpinning the family systems theory is the concept of the family life cycle (Carter and McGoldrick, 1980). This is seen as a matrix of critical stages, starting with the beginning of a family and continuing until its dissolution. Within this are key transitional phases. In the field of death and dying, the concept of the family life cycle is seen as increasingly important (Smith, 1990) and used as a framework in sociological studies (Finch and Wallis, 1993; Zlatin, 1995). Using 'life course' as a theoretical framework, and focusing on inheritance and wills, Finch and Wallis (1993) interviewed 99 people to find out the extent to which material relationships can promote or fracture personal bonds between family members when death occurs. No firm conclusions were drawn, although the authors were keen to emphasise the potential value of using life course from a conceptual perspective. Zlatin (1995) interviewed eight patients with incurable cancer, using the notion of life themes to elicit their understanding of their illness. While recognising the limitations of her preliminary study, Zlatin concluded that using a framework of life themes may help health care professionals to understand how patients interpret their illness and, in so doing, explain the coping mechanisms used.

These studies indicate that death and dying are increasingly seen as critical events in the cyclical transitions of family systems and may often force the dying person and members of their family to reorganise and redefine relationships, particularly when death involves a parent or a young person. More importantly, the belief systems of families are seen by some investigators as the key to understanding how traditions, myths, legends, shared assumptions, expectations and prejudices are amalgamated within 'family scripts' (Burham, 1990). Thus, the health care professional's approach and manner in supporting patients' and families' experiences of death and dying is potentially a powerful one. In passing on beliefs and patterns of behaviour within families, they may, in turn, contribute to overall values and attitudes to death and the dying at a societal level.

Summary

The experience of dying is multidimensional and involves people in a range of physical, psychological, social, philosophical and spiritual responses. It is clear that the experience of dying in contemporary western society has been shaped by technological advances in medicine. The physical aspects of a lingering death have a profound impact on bodily function and invariably affect quality of life. Despite improvements in pain relief and symptom management which serve to alleviate much physical suffering, dying involves the person facing the death of the self.

Various strategies appear to be used as part of the process of psychological coping. How people cope also appears to be related to the care and support provided at a social level. This care has traditionally been provided by family members, but increasingly much of the care has shifted to professionals in institutions, giving rise to an institutionalised death system. This shift exposes professional carers, in particular nurses, to various aspects of the dying process, as nurses comprise the predominant group of health care professionals involved in caring for the dying.

THE EXPERIENCE OF NURSES WHO CARE FOR DYING INDIVIDUALS

'The patient's growing awareness of her fate contributed to the increasing intolerance of staff. Her growing need to prepare herself for death was cause for more rebuff. Mrs Abel did find in the night nurse someone who would respond to her plea: "I want somebody to love me." The nurse, whose own mother had died of cancer, felt a reawakening of this personal loss and, holding Mrs Abel in her arms, let her cry out. But this form of comfort care so usual in dying situations was soon given up by this nurse. She, too, avoided and isolated Mrs Abel, using the typical strategy of sending an aide into the room when Mrs Abel called. The nurse wished also to heavily sedate Mrs Abel but could not because of her slow respiration. Mrs Abel would awaken and scream at night, disturbing other patients and the sentimental order of the ward. Clearly this unusually upsetting behaviour had to be stopped, by discharging the patient.'

(Strauss and Glaser 1970, p.167)

The impact on the nurse of caring for dying patients was vividly illustrated by Strauss and Glaser (1970, p.167) in the above extract from *Anguish — A Case History of a Dying Trajectory*. Mrs Abel, a patient with cancer, died slowly. As her story highlights, there are multiple needs and dimensions in the experience of dying. Nurses who care for the dying are placed daily alongside people who have to live with losses. How nurses respond to, and cope with, the grief and distress of people facing death is of great importance, not only for the nurses themselves but also because of its effect on patients and their family.

In the following sections, the concepts and relationship between nursing and caring are explored from a generic nursing perspective. This generic approach is necessary because these concepts underpin almost every branch of nursing, including the care of the dying. It is followed by a section focusing specifically on the impact of death and dying on nurses, and on the involvement of nurses with the dying. These issues are important within the context of care provided by nurses to dying people and establishing nurse-patient relationships and will form an integral part of the study of the cases in this study and their analysis.

Nursing and caring

The primary goals of nursing are promoting and restoring health, preventing illness and caring for the sick (Watson, 1985). The act of nursing involves a person delivering care to another person.

The delivery of care may take many forms, ranging from being alongside someone, described as presencing, to listening, performing and advocating. The concept of caring has been highlighted therefore as central to nursing (Watson, 1985; Leininger, 1986; Benner and Wrubel, 1989). Caring is seen as relational and rooted within nurse-patient interactions, giving rise to a relationship where people are engaged in giving and receiving help.

In recent years the nature of caring, and the extent to which caring is embedded in nursing, has generated much discussion (Dunlop, 1986; Leininger, 1988; Smith, 1990; McMahon and Pearson, 1992; Kitson, 1993). In particular, the nature of caring for dying people has remained important. This is exemplified by the works of early religious nursing sisters who tended to poor, sick and dying people who would otherwise not have received care.

Today, notions of care and caring continue to be of prime significance, particularly in the case of terminally ill patients. As a person's disease advances and cure is no longer the goal, the disease-modifying therapies diminish in importance, and care that was initially curative in its goal changes to care that is palliative. In the latter, the goal of care is to achieve the best quality of life for patients and their families by providing relief from pain and other distressing symptoms and offering a support system that integrates physical, psychological, social and spiritual aspects of care (World Health Organization, 1990).

The literature on caring can be divided into three areas: studies that explore caring from a conceptual perspective, those that attempt to clarify the components of caring, and those that seek to analyse the relationship between nurses and patients. The word 'care' originates from the Old English *carian*, meaning to trouble oneself (Dunlop, 1986). Caring has been expressed as helping another grow and actualise himself/herself. It is a way of relating to someone that involves development, in the same way that friendship can only emerge through mutual trust and a deepening and qualitative transformation of the relationship (Mayeroff, 1971; Kitson, 1985). Others have suggested that caring is a form of loving (Ray, 1981; Campbell, 1984; Jacono, 1993). McFarlane (1988) proposes that genuine affection, friendship and even love are present in nursing but argues that it is fundamentally the love as seen in *charitas* or *agape* which constitutes the basic motivational force for caring.

Like the terms death and dying, the construction of care is related to the use and interpretation of language (Dunlop, 1986; Marks-Maran, 1992). Marks-Maran (1992, p.99) pointed out that, if caring is defined as in the phrase 'to take care of', it implies a position of control and power over another. This becomes problematic, particularly when care is delivered from a paternalistic stance. Caring can also be defined as 'to care for' someone, which may imply a degree of sympathetic involvement. In contrast, 'to care about' someone implies a deeper involvement and it is about 'feeling *with* another person, rather than feeling for another' (Marks-Maran, 1992). Griffin (1983) expanded on the notion of caring by stating that caring is an interpersonal process and incorporates two primary domains: nurses' attitudes and emotions, and the activities that nurses engage in while carrying out nursing functions.

Implicit within these expressions of caring are the qualities of relating, awareness, trust and a sense of human value. Similar expressions of caring can be seen in other works (Benner, 1984; 1985; Gaut, 1986; Muetzel, 1988).

While such expressions appear to capture the essence of caring, particularly in nursing, the interpretation and translation of the concept to nursing practice remains contentious. This is, in part, dependent on the views of how caring is constructed and located within the structures of the nurse-patient relationship.

A limited number of studies have attempted to identify the components of caring from the perspectives of nurses (James, 1986; Wolf, 1986; Davis and Oberle, 1990; Hull, 1991; Morrison, 1991; Smith, 1992), patients (Larson, 1984; Brown, 1986; Mayer, 1986; Cronin and Harrison, 1988) and other primary caregivers (Skorupha and Bohnet, 1982; Ryan, 1992). Smith (1992) highlighted the failure of nursing leaders to appreciate and conceptualise the complexity of the notion of caring beyond the level of initial definitions. According to Graham (1983), James (1989), and Smith (1992), those qualities used in caring, such as feelings of concern, empathy, and love are demanding and constitute 'emotion work'. Smith's study (1992, p.136) showed that nurses are involved not only in the emotional work with patients in delivering care but also 'have to work emotionally on themselves in order to appear to care, irrespective of how they personally feel about themselves, their patients, or their conditions and circumstances'. And although as difficult and taxing as physical labour, emotional labour is often unrecognised and undervalued, primarily because it is readily dismissed as 'women's domestic work' (James 1986; 1989). In her study, James found that nurses in a hospice, while not underestimating the value of emotional work in good care, would often understate the emotional labour of their tasks. James coined the term 'carework' to refer to the nursing care of the dying, in part to include the emotional labour that is required of nurses who care for the dying.

Evidence from research studies conducted on nurses found that caring behaviours identified by them include listening and talking and allowing for expression of feelings and touching (Larson, 1986; 1987; Wolf, 1986; Forrest, 1989; Geissler, 1990). In general, nurses have tended to focus on affective and psychosocial components as the most desirable indicators of caring (for reviews, see Morse, Solberg, Neander et al, 1990; Hull, 1991). This contrasts directly with some studies on patients' perceptions of caring behaviours which identified clinical competence and attention to physical care as indicative of caring behaviours (Larson, 1984; Mayer, 1986; Cronin and Harrison, 1988). Constructs of caring have steadily emerged from recent studies, and these have been argued as potentially important, particularly in providing the basis for investigations into nurse-patient relationships (Morse, 1991; Christensen, 1993). For instance, Muetzel

(1988) identified the concepts of partnership, reciprocity and intimacy as major components of nurse-patient encounters and the interactions from these three concepts provide the atmosphere, dynamics and the spirit of that encounter between people.

In recent decades there has been an increase in the literature that alludes to the nature of nurse-patient relationships. Discussions have centred on the therapeutic and non-therapeutic nature of nursing (McMahon and Pearson, 1992), responses of nurses to the types and personalities of patients (Stockwell, 1972; Kelly and May, 1982; Smith 1992), and the importance of communication in successful interaction with patients (Buckmann, 1988; Wilkinson, 1991). Much of this discussion is an off-shoot of a wider debate about nursing, particularly in relation to redressing the traditional imbalance, which placed values on physical care and task performance at the expense of meeting psychological, social and spiritual needs. While this literature is constructive because it has provided information for establishing and developing nurse-patient relationships, it is only recently that the types and characteristics of nurse-patient relationships have been investigated.

Several studies have identified levels and depths of nurse-patient relationships (Forest, 1989; Morse, 1991; Morse et al, 1992; Ramos, 1992). Morse et al (1992) showed that nurses use different levels of engagement with patients and the level of engagement is affected by factors such as whether the focus of the engagement is placed on the nurse or on the patient, and whether the response elicited from the nurse is learned or reflexive (arising from within the self). These authors showed that constant exposure to the suffering of patients is emotionally draining. Although, initially, suffering evokes reflexive, spontaneous expressions of verbal comfort (sympathy, compassion, pity — termed the first-level reflexive response), in the long term these expressions are replaced by alternative methods of engagement in order to exercise control. These include the use of first-level reflected response (for example, labelling or distancing), a professional second-level response (such as the use of therapeutic empathy), or the use of detached, second-level responses (false assurances, rote behaviours).

Other studies (Morse, 1991; Ramos, 1992) have drawn attention to the varied and dynamic nature of nurse-patient relationships. Clinical, therapeutic, connected or over-involved relationships have all been identified, depending on the depth, duration and levels of contact between the nurse and patient (Morse, 1991). Morse highlighted the interplay and covert negotiations that operate before a relationship of mutual satisfaction is reached. More recently, Christensen's (1993) study on nursing partnership incorporated both patients' and nurses' perspectives and showed that creating a partnership involves discrete elements of 'work' from both patient and nurse, affected mainly by a process of 'passage' during hospitalisation.

These empirical studies have yielded important information about how nurses are involved or not involved in relationships with patients. This involvement highlights the essence of the relationship by identifying focus of control and determining the balance and power of relationships. While these investigations may contribute to an understanding of some specific issues confronting nurses when entering relationships, the following questions remain to be answered: what is the nature of involvement between the nurse and the dying person (and their families)? How do nurses cope with the continual impact on themselves of death and the processes of dying?

Involvement of nurses with dying individuals and their families

A death profoundly affects members of the immediate family and close friends as well as health care professionals. The reactions and behaviours of family members, friends and carers towards the dying person may affect how that person responds to their situation. A small number of studies have begun to explore the nature of emotional involvement of nurses with dying patients and their immediate families.

As shown in Field's (1984) and more recently Samarel's (1991) and James' (1993) studies, it is clear that nurses find it difficult to care and, at the same time, remain emotionally uninvolved with patients. Emotional involvement has traditionally been identified as an unavoidable aspect of caring for the dying, particularly by those working in hospices. Moreover, an emotional involvement underpins much of the caring behaviour identified in a decade of studies (Castles and Murray, 1979; Skorupha and Bohnet, 1982; McGinnis, 1986; Davis and Oberle, 1990; Ryan, 1992). In particular, Ryan (1992) showed that being honest, staying with the patient during difficult times and providing a helping-trusting relationship was highly valued by patients' care-givers and hospice nurses. From their interviews of 126 patients and nurses in six institutions, Castles and Murray (1979) concluded that working with the dying evokes intense personal feelings, and it is important for staff to recognise the range and intensity of positive and negative feelings. The authors cautioned against the continued investment in this intensity, arguing that the phenomenon of death saturation is real and there are personal limits of tolerance.

In their study on the supportive role of nurses in palliative care, Davis and Oberle (1990) highlighted that the essence of emotional involvement lies in the giving of self. Caring for the dying involves being alongside them and being exposed to individual vulnerabilities that are specific to dying, which are often not met in normal circumstances (see Chapter 8). This work is performed in a subtle way, or is not articulated (Duke and Copp 1991). Davis and Oberle suggested the following 'special features' of nursing work with the dying:

- 'valuing': respecting others and the patient as individuals;

- 'connecting': establishing and continuing a good relationship with the family;

- 'empowering': facilitating strengths within the family by encouraging and defusing;

- 'doing for': enabling the patient by controlling pain and resolving problems;

- 'finding meaning': helping to focus on living and acknowledging death;

- 'preserving own integrity': valuing oneself as a nurse and being aware of one's own needs and attachments.

While the authors imply that these features define the role of the specialist nurse, they are just as likely to be experienced in general nursing work and so do not appear to be exclusive to those who work with the dying.

In contrast, two UK nurse investigators (James, 1986; Smith, 1992), recognising the importance of emotional work in 'caring', have focused on exploring the feelings of nurses who care for dying patients. These studies were the first of their kind in the UK to show explicitly the nature of emotional involvement in caring for the dying. Smith (1992) identified several patient care situations to illustrate the depth of nurses' attachments and non-attachments to dying patients and highlighted the different strategies used by nurses to manage and package deaths. Smith also explored the feelings that are involved in this area of care. She highlighted that some student nurses felt cheated when patients they had been caring for died when they were off duty. This feeling was intensified when ward staff failed to let the students know of the deaths. Smith related the feeling of being cheated to the lack of opportunity to conclude the care that the student had begun. Some nurses see performing last offices for the person who has died as part of completing care. The act of closure appears important and will be considered further in Chapter 8.

In an earlier study on the work of nurses in a hospice, James (1986) also found that nurses used several strategies to manage their feelings when caring for the dying. The more mature, older staff had thought about their own deaths, and most nurses used their own life experiences in empathising with patients' feelings. On occasion, the lack of a clear lead in how to approach conversations with patients, who may or may not have been ready to talk about their impending deaths, also posed a difficulty for the nurses. As in Smith's (1992) study, nurses in James's (1986) study also talked about their need to know what happened when a patient died if they were not on duty at the time. Some even looked in the *in memoriam* columns of the local press. In conclusion, it seems that the studies of Smith and James capture the essence of nursing the dying to a much greater extent than Davis and Oberle (1990).

In hospices, the encouragement and value placed on families and patients as units of care make the direct involvement of nurses with family members an explicit part of care. Studies conducted on families have focused primarily on identifying their needs and evaluating the nursing care provided to them (for a review, see Wilson-Barnett and Richardson, 1993). These studies gathered information from families rather than nurses and have provided some insights into those nursing actions or behaviours that are perceived as helpful. These include providing information about aspects of patient care and treatment, teaching families about the signs of imminent death, permitting free visiting of the patient and having staff visits at home (Skorupka and Bonnet, 1982; Garland et al, 1984). Clinical competence was also seen as important, particularly involving pain relief (Wright and Dyck, 1984; McGinnis, 1986; Hull, 1990).

A few studies have yielded information on the emotional aspects of nurses' behaviours in connection with enabling families to air their feelings. An early investigation showed that families found least supportive those nursing behaviours that encouraged the airing of feelings (Freihofer and Felton, 1976). In fact, the families did not want attention to be focused on them, but Hull's (1990) more recent study obtained contrasting findings. Hull concluded that whether or not nursing behaviours are helpful in this area is dependent on the need of individual families to maintain control of their feelings. Consequently, to encourage expression of feelings in families that need to maintain control would be seen as unsupportive and distressful, whereas families who want to discuss their feelings would perceive the ability of nurses to provide this support as helpful.

Another aspect of involvement with families relates to focus of attention. When a patient's condition deteriorates, families may still want to be involved in care-giving but they expect less attention for themselves (Wilson-Barnett and Richardson, 1993). This is an interesting phenomenon because it is common in nursing to find that nurses shift their attention to relatives as imminent death approaches (see Chapter 8). An understanding of this discrepancy between families' expectations and nurses' behaviours may help nurses be more aware of different levels of involvement during the process of engaging and disengaging with patients and relatives.

Clearly, an important feature of the relationship between nurses, patients and their families is that eventually the involvement with the patient and family members comes to an end when the patient dies or, as in most hospices, following a period of support to families in their bereavement. Davies and Oberle (1990) call this ending 'breaking the connection'. This phenomenon may be seen as an important aspect of emotional involvement, particularly in the way nurses accommodate grief and transitions in the course of their professional work. Unfortunately, there is a dearth of literature on this aspect of nurses' experience.

Impact of death and dying on nurses

Professionals, as people, will at some point have to die and confront issues of mortality. Questions have been raised by a number of authors regarding the impact on them of continued exposure to dying people (Vachon, 1978; Stedeford, 1988). For instance, what effect does long-term work with dying persons and exposure to death have on the professional? How do professionals cope with this impact? These questions seem particularly relevant to nurses who have chosen to work in hospice settings, as well as in A&E departments, where traumas and incidents of death and dying are common. Despite the intrinsic interest of these questions, any attempt at an answer would require a study design different from this one, so this issue will not be explored further.

Various studies have been undertaken to explore the processes of dying and death on nurses. Most nurses will readily supply anecdotal accounts to highlight the uncertainty, fear, anxiety and guilt experienced in dealing with dying and death. These accounts have been substantiated by more systematic studies (Bram and Katz, 1989; Alexander and Ritchie, 1990). For instance, there is evidence that students and registered nurses find caring for dying people stressful and often experience feelings of inadequacy and inability, particularly in coping with pain management and symptom control (Hockley, 1989; Copp and Dunn, 1993; Corner, 1993; Copp, 1994). Although education, by increasing nursing skills and knowledge of pain and symptom management, appears crucial in enabling feelings of helplessness to be overcome, nurses are seldom provided with opportunities to express feelings generated by death experiences in the course of work (Castles and Murray, 1979; Smith, 1992).

The relationship between unresolved personal feelings about death and dying and the use of defence mechanisms has been investigated in a number of studies (Kniesel, 1968; Phillips, 1972). These defence behaviours include the use of technical language, avoidance of contact with the dying person and using bed numbers and disease when referring to the patient (Bowers, 1975; Gow, 1982; Maguire, 1985). Menzies (1960) pointed out that nursing systems incorporate features of detachment, ritualisation of tasks, depersonalisation, categorisation and denial of feelings into everyday care which have the effect of protecting the nurse from anxiety-provoking situations. Contacts with patients in hospitals were purposely split into lists of tasks, each allocated to an individual nurse as a defence strategy against anxiety.

Given that working with dying patients is stressful, it is unsurprising to find that some studies have attempted to identify the motivations and coping strategies of nurses who pursue this type of work. These studies, conducted on nurses in hospices, have focused predominantly on four key areas: motivations and personality, identifying stressors, manifestation of stress and coping strategies (for a review, see Vachon, 1986). Although research in hospice nursing tends to be sparse, there is evidence to suggest that a need for emotional reward plays a major part in motivation to work in hospices. Other motivations include a desire for mastery over death, intellectual appeal, affiliation with a charismatic leader, a sense of calling and previous personal experience. However, for some, entry into hospice nursing was simply by accident or convenience (Vachon, 1978), although a more recent study (Rasmussen et al, 1995) showed that inexperienced nurses embarking on hospice work for the first time were motivated by the desire to have an opportunity to form close relationships with patients and families. Most of the nurses in this study had previous experience of relatives dying in an undignified way. The desire of these nurses to 'give of themselves and/or grow as a person' were strong motivators.

It has also been shown that hospice nurses tend to be more independent, creative and religious than hospital nurses, who are more practical in their approach to work (Amenta, 1984). Earlier studies also showed that hospice nurses who are timid or shy tend to leave after a few months (Lyall et al, 1976; 1980). Subsequent studies have attempted to identify the types of stressors that nurses experience when caring for dying people. These include aspects of teamwork, such as communication and support, and the struggle between the democratic hospice atmosphere and the traditional hierarchical hospital structure, and would seem to be similar to stressors experienced by nurses in other settings. However, what emerged as specific to hospice care were the rapid succession of deaths, the lack of emotional readiness in handling emotional situations and frustrations with inadequacies in dealing with pain (for a review, see Vachon, 1993).

There is also some evidence from James's (1986) study that nurses cope with numerous deaths by remembering individuals rather than collective numbers. According to James, nurses collect and store a repertoire of patient memories that may comprise a collection of stories about particular people, their dignified deaths, idiosyncrasies and brave families. The enormity of the number of deaths only became apparent when nurses in the study began reflecting on the deaths they had handled in the previous year. James (1986, p.311) stated that: 'The dying at Byresfold and the deaths were disturbing. They were optimised, minimised, routinised and dealt with in a variety of "standard" ways, but each time they caused some disruption. In nursing the dying it is inevitable that individual and collective defence mechanisms will evolve as nurses distance themselves from the full implications of a death, but what is important is the form that such "protection" takes. In the end most of the nurses felt there was a time to go.'

Vachon (1986) showed that, contrary to popular belief, long-term involvement with dying patients does not result in greater stress when compared with short-term involvement, such as that experienced in A&E, obstetric and intensive care units. Nurses in these units experienced more stress due to frustrations about the lack of time available to meet the needs of patients and families in accomplishing a good death.

Data from interviews conducted with nurses in Field's (1984) study showed that they found unexpected deaths more difficult to cope with. The findings of both Vachon's (1986) and Field's studies contrast with Glaser's and Strauss's (1968) work, in which the authors found the opposite effect. In Glaser and Strauss's study, staff found patients who died quickly and unexpectedly easier to cope with than those who took a long time to die. There may be variations in the perception of what dying and death means to individual nurses, to the extent to which this matches their individual view of how they would wish to die. However, perhaps the most important factor is that, with time, there has been an increasing shift in health care culture towards increased openness when caring for the dying and in forming nurse-patient relationships. This tends to promote coping in nurses with regard to anticipated deaths as reflected in the more recent studies and may account for the different findings of the studies published in 1970s and 1980s.

Without further analysis, information about how nurses cope with death remains limited. Until more investigations are undertaken, the long-term impact on nurses who are exposed to death and dying is still relatively unclear, despite emphasis being placed by hospices on the need to balance work with leisure and family activities as part of coping.

Summary

The experience of nursing is clearly rooted in the concept of care and the process of delivering that care. Central to these notions are relational constructs that involve people in different levels and depths of engagement in the nurse-patient relationship. A few exploratory studies have examined the involvement and motivation of nurses engaged in the care of those facing impending death. This has mostly focused on nurses in palliative care/hospice nursing. Because of the multiple needs of the dying person, the focus and scope of these studies vary. It is clear that nurses use a range of strategies and mechanisms to negotiate, develop and maintain relationships with patients and families. The depth and levels of involvement vary and, depending on the individuals concerned, issues of emotion, personality and focus of control may be of greatest importance. Recently, a distinction has been drawn between the physical and emotional labour of care, particularly when nursing the dying. The effects of short- and long-term involvement of nurses with dying patients are still poorly understood, although there is an indication that recall, in terms of collective numbers of deaths, may have an impact on nurses who are continually exposed to death.

2. Current theories of death and dying

Several theoretical frameworks on death and dying have been postulated during the past three decades (Glaser and Strauss, 1965; Kübler-Ross, 1969; Pattison, 1977; Corr, 1992; Buckman, 1993). Seminal works such as those of Kübler-Ross (1969) and Glaser and Strauss (1965) challenged the approach and care given by health care professionals to those facing impending death. At the same time, both in the USA and the UK, the works of several other investigators such as Sudnow (1967), Weisman (1967; 1972), Hinton (1963; 1966) and Saunders (1959; 1967; 1972) sustained the general discussion on the care of the dying.

Central to the theories postulated during the 1960s and early 1970s is their focus on situations in practice, in particular, dying and deaths in institutions. Apart from Kübler-Ross' (1969) work, these earlier studies were mostly from the perspective of health care professionals. Kübler-Ross's 'stage theory' was arguably the most popular and well-known at the time. It continues to be popular today, despite recent criticisms and more contemporary theories (Corr, 1992; Buckman, 1993).

STAGE THEORY OF DYING

The five-stage model of dying

Until recently, Kübler-Ross's five-stage theory has been the principal model for coping with dying. Drawing on interviews with over 200 dying patients, Kübler-Ross postulated five stages in the process of psychological response to dying: denial, anger, bargaining, depression, and acceptance (Fig 1). According to this theory, the dying person initially reacts to the shock of news of an incurable illness by refusing to believe that it is true, thus denying the situation. This is followed by the second and third stages of anger and bargaining. In the latter stage, the person may engage in bargaining with God, for instance by making promises to God in exchange for more time to live. This is followed by depression when it becomes clear that they can no longer deny the progression of the disease. The fifth stage, acceptance, may occur if sufficient time and help are given to enable the person to work through their grief and sense of loss.

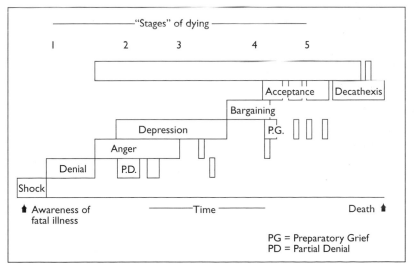

Fig 1 Five-stage model of dying (Kübler-Ross, 1969)

Reproduced with the kind permission of Simon & Schuster from *On Death and Dying* by Elisabeth Kubler-Ross. © 1969 by Elisabeth Kubler-Ross

The concept of stages stems from childhood developmental theory and has widespread appeal in providing an orderly sequence to the unfolding of human experiences during dying (Rainey, 1988). Kastenbaum (1985) discussed the reasons for the initial uncritical acceptance of this theory by health professionals and the general public by drawing attention to the following:

- The stage theory of dying reawakened and legitimised the topic of death which had previously been taboo for many people.

- The theory became, for many, the first exposure to systematic description of the death process.

- The theory reduced anxiety for professionals by providing a coherent, orderly structure to dying, which had been previously perceived as a vague, terrifying and overpowering entity.

In other words, Kübler-Ross's model gained acceptance largely because it filled a void in health care theory. However, questions have been raised about the adequacy and validity of the stage theory (Weisman, 1974; Charmaz, 1980; Feigenberg, 1980; Kastenbaum, 1985; Corr, 1992). The internal validity of Kübler-Ross' data analysis has been criticised, as has the absence of any description of her sample or definition of terms used. Probably the most important criticism relates to the fact that the stage theory assumes too mechanistic an approach, with the dying person moving through the universal five stages.

Although Kübler-Ross cautioned that a dying patient should not be rushed through the stages, there nevertheless appears to be an implicit suggestion in the theory that a valued destination can be achieved — that is, acceptance. The descriptive element of the theory is therefore sometimes misinterpreted as prescriptive, to the extent that some health professionals have tried to move dying patients through the five stages (Pattison, 1977; Rainey, 1988). However, there has been no evidence from clinical practice to support this unidirectional movement of the dying process. In fact, experience suggests that dying patients oscillate between periods of calm, fear, hope, depression, anger, sadness and withdrawal. These reactions occur in various combinations and at varying times (Buckman, 1993).

Corr (1992) also criticised the stage theory because it focuses solely on psychosocial dynamics to the exclusion of physical and, to a lesser extent, spiritual dimensions. The theory's emphasis is on defence mechanisms and responses to threat and conflict. As a theoretical model on dying it appears limited, therefore, given the multifaceted elements of dying and death.

A three-stage model of the process of dying

Buckman (1993) proposed the three stage model (Fig 2) in an attempt to redress some of the perceived flaws in Kübler-Ross's five-stage model.

Fig 2. Three-stage model of dying (Buckman, 1993)

Initial stage ('facing the threat')	Chronic stage ('being ill')	Final stage ('acceptance')

A mixture of reactions which are characteristic of the individual and which may include any, or all, of the following:
  Fear
  Anxiety
  Shock
  Disbelief
  Anger
  Denial
  Guilt
  Humour
  Hope/despair
  Bargaining
	1. Resolution of those elements of the initial response which are resolvable
	
	2. Diminution of intensity of all emotions ('monochrome state')
		1. Defined by the patient's acceptance of death
		
		2. Not an essential state provided that the patient is not distressed, is communicating normally and is making decisions normally

Reproduced with the kind permission of Oxford University Press from *Communication in Palliative Care: A practical guide* by R. Buckman, in The Oxford Textbook of Palliative Medicine by Doyle, D., Hanks, G.W., MacDonald, N. (Eds), 1997.

Buckman, argued that, when confronted with impending death, people react in a way consistent with their character and the way they have coped with difficulties in the past. Thus, patients' reactions are not a product of the stage in process or the diagnosis. Buckman further argues that it is more useful to perceive a patient's emotions as sources of insight into their personality, rather than as indicators of the stage they are passing through. Furthermore, such emotions are 'mosaic' in form and very likely to occur simultaneously, and not with serial transition, as suggested by Kübler-Ross. Buckman further pointed out that several emotions and responses, in particular fear of dying, guilt, hope, despair and humour, are not included in Kübler-Ross's five-stage system, even though they are commonly seen in clinical practice.

Two central principles form the basis of Buckman's (1993) argument for his three-stage model. First, the mixture of emotions and responses exhibited by a person facing death are characteristic of the person and not of the diagnosis or the stage of the dying process. Second, during the process of dying, the person's progress is marked by resolving the elements of those emotions that are resolvable and not by a change in the type of emotions.

As shown in Fig 2, the model incorporates an initial stage, a chronic stage and a final stage. Buckman lists 11 emotions in the initial stage and states that a person can be considered to have entered the chronic stage when elements of the initial emotions have resolved, with or without assistance. The chronic stage may or may not occur, depending on whether the person resolves their emotions. If this does not happen, the chronic stage does not exist for the person, and Buckman advises the professional dealing with such a patient to seek help for them. In the third and final stage, the patient appears to experience less emotional intensity, and this is defined by acceptance of the impending death, although acceptance is not perceived to be an absolute necessity.

One of the strengths of Buckman's model lies in its constructive attempt to redress many of the criticisms levied against Kübler-Ross' model. It provides a refreshing change and contrast to the usual criticisms of Kübler-Ross, which are not accompanied by constructive suggestions. Buckman has addressed many of the limitations of the model, such as seeing emotions exhibited as sources of a person's characteristics, rather than 'stage-bound'. However, as a theoretical model, Buckman's own still faces many of the criticisms levied against a stage-based approach. In particular, it falls into the trap of appearing mechanistic at the general or macro-level. In addition, the emphasis of the model, like that of Kübler-Ross, is based solely on emotions and reactions and, as such, is unidimensional. Nevertheless, as Buckman (1993, p.51) states: 'It does seem that an alternative framework can be put forward which more accurately reflects the dying patient's progress and which will allow the professional greater power of analysis and prediction.'

The context of awareness theory

In contrast to and preceding the stage theories, Glaser and Strauss (1965) used a sociological approach to analyse the awareness of dying in hospitals. Using participant observations and interviews, the authors collected data from three hospitals. Their analyses on the interactions between hospital staff and patients with life-threatening illnesses led them to describe four contexts of awareness between hospital staff and patients: closed awareness, suspicion awareness, mutual pretence awareness and open awareness.

Closed awareness occurs when staff know of the patient's poor prognosis but do not share this information. Glaser and Strauss (1965) reported that nurses and doctors engage in conversations that circumvent disclosure, keep conversations to the minimum and steer away from conversations about the future, especially when a patient is thought certain to die within days. This initial level of awareness invariably changes; patients may move to either suspicion awareness or to full awareness of their prognosis.

Suspicion awareness is seen as an unstable situation in which the patient begins to suspect the seriousness of his condition. He may then attempt to confirm his suspicion directly or indirectly, such as by sneaking a look at medical records or making direct inquiries of the staff. Alternatively, he may initiate 'confirmation-seeking tactics' about his condition, inducing staff to adopt different strategies in response. These may include measures aimed at further preventing the patient from knowing the truth by actively controlling facial and body mannerisms, for example, when dealing with the patient.

Glaser and Strauss (1965) described suspicion awareness as being a 'fantastic psychological strain' for families, staff and patient. The consequence may be that the patient will die without ever knowing the truth, although in some cases he may eventually move to full awareness of the condition. Here, a 'mutual pretence' may arise, particularly when staff and patient both know that the patient is dying but choose to pretend that he is going to live. In contrast, when both staff and patient know and choose to acknowledge that the patient is dying, open awareness results. However, this situation is by no means an easy one. It is fraught with uncertainties and ambiguities, giving rise to divergent expectations of 'appropriate dying'. In particular, tension can exist when the patients' style of dying contradicts staff expectations.

Dying trajectories

Two years after the publication of *Awareness of Dying*, Glaser and Strauss (1968) published *Time for Dying*. The authors hypothesised that there is a relationship between the phases of dying and several death expectations, or trajectories. These trajectories were:

(i)   certain death at a known time;
(ii) certain death at an unknown time;
(iii) uncertain death but a known time when the certainty will be established;
(iv) uncertain death and an unknown time when the question will be resolved.

The authors proposed that an individual's dying trajectory comprises two important elements — time and shape. This means that specific dying trajectories vary in duration and form. For instance, the course of dying may be rapid, slow, or it may plateau. It may also move up or down (with short-term improvements and relapses) before finally plunging downwards. Conflicts and tensions in patient, family and staff occur when an expected death trajectory changes, with interruption of organisational work, for instance, if a patient unexpectedly dies or continues to linger on when a swift death is expected. Using some of the concepts from these two major works to illustrate the course of dying in hospital, Strauss and Glaser (1970) presented *Anguish: A Case History of a Dying Trajectory* based on the experiences of Mrs Abel, a patient with cancer who exemplified a lingering dying trajectory. This case history provided detailed, rich accounts of the experiences of a woman and the nurses involved in her care and demonstrates one of the four proposed death trajectories — the concept of certain death at an unknown time.

In analysing Glaser and Strauss's works it appears that a major strength of both studies lies in their immersion in everyday realities. As such, the theories remain relevant in contemporary hospitals. The most significant impact of their work by far is their influence on health care professionals' approach to communication and interactions with the dying. In particular, their work provides the basis for subsequent studies and research into the disclosure of bad news to patients and families. The two studies (including the case history of Mrs Abel) also provide useful insight into behaviours and responses of patients, families, doctors and nurses when faced with the process of dying.

As theoretical models Glaser and Strauss's substantive theories on dying provide the potential for further theory development. Nevertheless, the weakness of the theories are perhaps the lack of a micro-analysis of several key issues. The reader is provided with broad, major themes at a descriptive level with few attempts to deepen the plausibility of some of the hypotheses. Also, the authors did not describe their sample and/or methods of analysis and, while it is stated that comparison groups were used to maximise differences and similarities, it is unclear what those groups were or how the comparison was undertaken.

The living-dying interval/phase theory of dying

Drawing on Glaser and Strauss's (1965, 1968) works, Pattison (1977) proposed the 'living-dying interval' model (Figs 3 and 4). Pattison stated that we all project ahead a trajectory of our lives. Based on experience from his clinical practice, he argued that this trajectory is changed when a crisis occurs, such as the knowledge of death. He defines the living-dying interval as that occurring between the 'crisis of the knowledge of death and the point of death'. There are three clinical phases in the living-dying interval: acute crisis phase, chronic living-dying phase and the terminal phase.

Pattison postulated that as carers our first task is to deal appropriately with the reactions presented by the patient so that the person's life does not disintegrate into chaos. For instance, it is not unusual to find psychological defence mechanisms being used, such as those described by

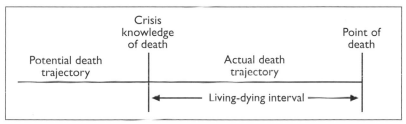

Fig 3 Living-dying interval (Pattison, 1977)

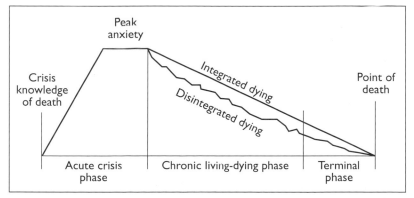

Fig 4 Phases of dying (Pattison, 1977)

Figs 3–5. Reproduced with the kind permission of Simon & Schuster from *The Experience of Dying* by E. Mansell Pattison. © 1977 by Prentice Hall Inc.

Kübler-Ross (1965) which include denial, anger and bargaining. According to Pattison, reducing anxiety by focusing on reality and providing emotional support are likely to help the dying person express appropriate emotional responses to their 'living-dying'.

The second task is to respond to the ways the person adapts to the chronic living-dying phase and, finally, the third task is to enable the person to move into the terminal phase. The onset of this phase is often not precise but is seen to begin when the dying person starts to withdraw from the outside world (Norton, 1963; Lieberman, 1965).

Overall, Pattison's living-dying interval model stems from a combination of psycho-dynamic and humanistic frameworks. Unlike other theories, his model takes into account the need for integrating dying according to the pace, feelings and reactions of the person. The strength of his work, therefore, is largely the result of being able to relate directly and meaningfully to everyday clinical experiences. As a theoretical model on death and dying it proposes several tentative hypotheses. For example, there is the assumption that, following the acute crisis phase, dying takes on either an integrated or disintegrated form depending on how the initial crisis phase is handled. However, a third form, lacking from Pattison's model, may also be envisaged in which both integrated and disintegrated dying occur at different times (Fig 5). Moreover, there is also the assumption that the process of dying is always a downward trend. This is clearly not the case, because many people may 'plateau' and then rapidly enter the terminal phase, as shown in Fig 5.

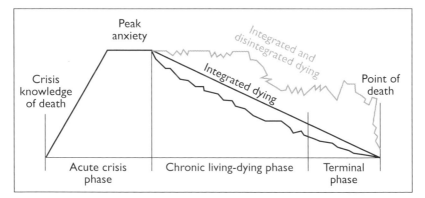

Fig 5 Integrated and disintegrated dying with plateau and declines at different times (modified after Pattison, 1977)

A TASK-BASED APPROACH TO COPING WITH DYING

Since Pattison's attempt to provide a framework for understanding the process of dying, interest in this area was dormant until recently. Corr (1992) argued that it is crucial to critically re-examine the usefulness of previous models and to draw on knowledge from allied disciplines (such as bereavement and human behaviour studies), in order to look afresh at how models guide our understanding. In the 1980s, many of the earlier works on the concept of coping and bereavement were being extended, with emphasis on research that is aimed at helping people cope better. Thus, bereavement studies during that period focused on the area of grief work, based on developmental theories, taking the approach that the bereaved need to be engaged in working on 'tasks' of grieving if they are to be successful in adjusting to their bereavement (Worden, 1991).

The underlying premise is that a bereaved person has to work on their grief, and this work, such as accepting the reality of the loss, working through the pain of grief, adjusting to an environment in which the deceased is missing and emotionally relocating the deceased and moving on with life essentially form the tasks of mourning. Recently, the underlying assumptions and long-standing beliefs that grief work is crucial for adjustment to bereavement have been challenged (Stroebe, 1992). In particular, emphasis has been placed on the failure of this hypothesis to take into account the complex interplay between confronting and inhibiting thoughts on loss and grief and their impact on health and well-being. Stroebe argued there may well be potential benefits in not confronting a loss.

The concept of 'tasks' was previously raised in Pattison's 'living-dying interval model'. It was originally conceived and discussed as a framework for understanding the process of dying from an individual's perspective (Kalish, 1979). In his chapter on 'the onset of the dying process', Kalish expounded on the tasks that confront the dying person, arguing that the realisation of impending death evokes both 'coping' and 'action' responses. For instance, the person may be increasingly motivated to deal with financial arrangements for the family, dealing with losses such as physical deterioration and family relationships. A decade after Kalish's notion of tasks of the dying person, Corr (1992) proposed a 'task-based approach to coping with dying' as a model for understanding the work of those who are dying and those who care for them. Operating on a similar basis to Kalish's initial thoughts on tasks, Corr's model featured two central concepts that were first identified by Kalish. These are the notions of tasks and coping with dying. Corr elaborated further by stating that individuals who are dying confront four primary areas of task work in coping:

- *physical* — satisfying bodily needs and minimising physical distress in ways that are consistent with other personal values;

- *psychological* — maximising psychological security, autonomy and richness of living;

- *social* — sustaining and enhancing interpersonal attachments of significance to the person and addressing social implications of dying;

- *spiritual* — the need to identify, develop and reaffirm sources of spiritual energy and, in so doing, foster hope.

While these are seen as important dimensions, in contrast to the notion of tasks, as set out in bereavement work, Corr was keen to point out that the task-based model operates from the perspective of individuals and their coping tasks. Corr asserts that this is because 'there is no single right way in which to cope with dying, although there may be better, worse, and even unacceptable modes of coping from the standpoint of each of those involved'. The second area of Corr's model lies in the notion of 'coping with dying'. Corr argues that coping takes various forms with various outcomes, depending on differing points of view. Nonetheless, Corr appears to base much of the conceptualisation of coping on the key works in the fields of coping and stress (Weisman, 1979; 1984; Lazarus and Folkman, 1984; Cooper, 1984). Corr states that 'coping encompasses more than just reacting to or defending against the events and challenges of life. Coping involves an awareness of events and challenges, plus efforts to contend with them.' A central underpinning of Corr's model lies in the basic premise that dying is not confined merely to the dying person. It affects all those who are drawn into the person's experience of dying, including family, friends and carers. And, because of its impact on carers, and because coping with dying involves not only awareness of events and challenges but also efforts to deal with them, Corr argued that, to be useful, any model must meet the following criteria: it should contribute to improved understanding, empowerment, participation and guidance for helpers to cope with dying. Corr subsequently argued that the 'task-based approach to a coping-with-dying model' fulfils these criteria.

The concept of tasks is therefore not a novel idea, and it is not surprising that this notion was adopted. Preparation for death, such as making provision for the family, has long been recognised as an important part of dying in pre-industrial and modern societies (Kellehear, 1993). Although Corr used the notion of tasks as a central underpinning of his model, it is clear that tasks serve a more fundamental function; it suggests active participation by the person dying and by those involved in helping them cope with dying. However, much of what Corr proposed is founded on the underlying assumption that tasks are central to the fundamental concerns of those dying. There have been no attempts to carry this analysis to deeper levels. For instance, commenting on Corr's model, Weisman (1992) and Kastenbaum and Thuell (1995) posed several questions. Weisman pointed out the need to examine in more depth the different tasks and sub-tasks related to coping — for instance, in the terminal phase. Issues that deserve further analysis include the relationship between dying and tasks and the nature and extent to which tasks might differ during dying, as opposed to those encountered in everyday life. These, together with the absence of empirical data to support his assertions, highlight the limitations of this model (Kastenbaum and Thuell, 1995).

Summary

The earlier theoretical frameworks on death and dying made significant contributions to clinical practice. In particular, they allowed health care professionals to re-examine their attitudes and behaviour towards dying patients and their families. This is exemplified by the growth of research on communication — for instance, with studies on how to break bad news and how to communicate with the dying and their families. Although the theories of dying clearly vary, depending on the approach adopted by the authors, there has been a gradual shift towards a more interactive and eclectic framework in recognition of the multifaceted nature of death and dying. This became most prominent in Corr's (1992) task-based model.

In the light of the theories and models on death and dying, it appears that the following must be considered when undertaking work in clinical practice and research:

- feelings and responses of individuals to death and dying, such as denial, anger and so on;

- interactions and interplays between the dying person and other individuals — mutual pretence, closed awareness, suspicion awareness;

- the form and duration (trajectory) of the dying process. An individual's dying may involve integrated or disintegrated dying, and is time-dependent: it may be slow, quick or may plateau. The process not only affects the individual who is dying but also others around him or her;

- the nature of the dimensions or tasks of dying. Dying people normally have to cope with four primary tasks of dying (physical, psychological, social and spiritual);

- the implications for carers. Improved understanding, empowerment, participation and guidance are seen as important for helpers in coping.

Some of the general limitations of the current theories are summarised here in order to highlight key areas for study.

First, as highlighted by Kastenbaum and Thuell (1995), none of the current theoretical approaches (Glaser and Strauss, 1965, 1968; Kübler-Ross, 1969; Pattison, 1977; Corr, 1992; Buckman, 1993) take full account of the dying individual's physical condition. The authors highlighted that the body as a physical reality, as an 'abode of the dying person' and consequently as a 'symbolic construction' that is created through interactions should comprise a salient part of any comprehensive theory of dying. Second, the dying person's own perspective is often unaccounted for in current theories. This omission has limited crucial understanding of the individual manner and styles of dying. Third, although Glaser and Strauss (1966) made important contributions, their work needs extension. For example, the shift towards a more 'open awareness' and 'truth-telling' culture may raise different problems for managing death and dying. The use of 'denial-like mechanisms' may thus take on a new meaning — for example, by becoming an important strategy for those facing imminent death within an increasingly open culture.

Fourth, although the sequential aspects of dying (dying trajectories and living-dying intervals) have been postulated in both Glaser and Strauss's (1968) and Pattison's (1977) works, several aspects of their postulations need to be extended and refined. For instance, the four death expectations or trajectories expounded by Glaser and Strauss (1968) (certain death at a known time; certain death at an unknown time; uncertain death but a known time when the certainty will be established; uncertain death and an unknown time when the question will be resolved) remain largely undeveloped. Given the growing interest in the care and management of people with life-threatening diseases, it appears important that the concept of 'certain death but at an unknown time' should be explored and developed further. Both Pattison (1977) and Glaser and Strauss (1968) showed that dying trajectories have a shape, form and duration. However, the nature of the form, shape and duration of dying has not subsequently been articulated in any depth.

Corr's (1992) task-based approach model has attempted to address some of the limitations of earlier theoretical propositions, such as the unidimensional approach (Kübler-Ross, 1969) by including the physical, psychological, social and spiritual aspects of dying and the relationships of dying individuals with carers. However, the lack of substantive study has limited its position as a theoretical framework. None the less, discussing the multidimensional aspects of dying, including responses of health care professionals, provides an important basis for further research.

3. Review of methods and tools used in studies on death and dying in health care settings

From the literature reviews in Chapters 1 and 2 it can be seen that a range of approaches have been used by investigators to answer questions on death and dying in health care settings. This chapter summarises the principal methods and tools that have been used in this field of research.

INTERVIEWS WITH DYING INDIVIDUALS

Formal, semistructured and informal interviews (Burgess, 1984; Ackroyd and Hughes, 1992) have been extensively used in qualitative and quantitative studies. These include works on the psychoanalytical aspects of dying (Cappon, 1959), physical and mental symptomatology of dying men and women (Hinton, 1963), influence of premorbid character traits (Hinton, 1966; 1971; 1975), and psychological reactions to dying (Kübler-Ross, 1969; Qvarnstrom, 1978). Most early studies stemmed from psychiatry and were generally medically oriented. In some studies interviews have been used to demonstrate the relationship between bodily illness and fantasy (Cappon, 1959), and to test for differences in the behaviours of patients with fatal illnesses and those with serious but not fatal illnesses (Witzel, 1975). A major criticism of these experiments is that they lack detailed description about the content of the interviews and the methods of data analysis.

More recently, studies using interviews have tended to focus on the experiences and meanings constructed by individuals facing death and cancer treatment (Castles and Murray, 1979; Schou, 1990; McLean, 1993). This was the approach of Castles and Murray (1979) who used semistructured interviews in the form of interview schedules to elicit responses from dying patients and nurses caring for them. They aimed to establish whether there was congruency between expected and observed behaviours of dying patients and their professional carers, including the kinds of nursing interventions that facilitate preferred behaviours in patients. This study was primarily a survey and, while the authors discussed the impact of organisational structures on care, the theoretical perspective about dying remained unclear.

PARTICIPANT OBSERVATION

Other studies have used participant observation (Burgess, 1984; Jorgensen, 1989; Ackroyd and Hughes, 1992) in combination with interviews (Glaser and Strauss, 1966; Sudnow, 1967; 1968; James, 1986; Field, 1987; 1989; Samarel, 1991). These were mainly conducted with nurses and other health professionals. Participant observation is traditionally a popular method in qualitative studies, as it provides the means for direct experiential and observational access to the insiders' world. For instance, Sudnow (1967), and Samarel (1991) used it in an ethnographic design as their method of choice to study the social context of dying in hospitals. Similarly, James (1986) used a combination of interviews with participant observation to observe nurses' work in a hospice.

Field's (1989) research used a symbolic-interactionist approach focusing on the care of the dying in acute hospitals and community. Although participant observation was used to gather data in part of the study, Field abandoned it owing to time constraints and adopted unstructured and informal interviews for the rest of his study. Glaser and Strauss' (1965; 1968) classic works used interviews and observations in their fieldwork to build substantive theory.

The use of systematic comparisons in the analysis of themes and categories from fieldwork have given rise to the method known as grounded theory.

However, the essence of this method is not stated explicitly but is implicit within the text of Glaser and Strauss' work. This often presents difficulties for novices attempting to use grounded theory methodology. Recently, the authors have produced books specifically on the procedures and techniques of grounded theory (Strauss, 1987; Strauss and Corbin, 1990) in an attempt to overcome this criticism.

It appears from this brief review that, apart from Castles and Murray (1979), most studies have focused either on patients or professionals. Few have explored the views of both.

QUESTIONNAIRES, PSYCHOLOGICAL TESTS AND PSYCHOLOGICAL AUTOPSY

Questionnaires and various psychological tests, such as death-anxiety scales, have been devised by psychologists (Boyar, 1964; Collett and Lester, 1969; Templer, 1970) and subsequently applied in health care settings (Cappon, 1962; Lieberman, 1965; Hoblit, 1972; Davis, 1973; Feifel, 1973; 1974; Carey, 1974). A particular interest has been on whether a dying person fears death more than a healthy person. However, the use of these techniques has been criticised on the basis that death anxiety is viewed as unidimensional, consisting of only a single type of fear or anxiety. Fulton (1961) argued that only the 'surface level' attitudes of subjects are seen using this approach and unconscious levels of death anxiety are not revealed (see also Schultz, 1978; Lester and Templer, 1993). An attempt to overcome this problem has used indirect methods, such as analysis of dream content (Handal and Rychlak, 1971) and imagery responses with the Rorschach inkblot test (Gordon, 1978). These approaches can show the presence of unconscious death anxiety and inner psyche in relation to dying.

Psychological 'autopsy', a method proposed by Weisman (1974), a US psychiatrist, uses a retrospective approach to reconstruct psychological and social aspects of a patient's dying process. Information is gathered from the interdisciplinary team members by performing a psychological autopsy on the deceased person (Weisman and Kastenbaum, 1968). This yields data on the 'experienced personal reactions' of deceased patients based solely on the perceptions and observations of health professionals and should, therefore, be viewed with caution. The lack of popularity of Weisman's method is also due to the very specialised techniques required.

CASE HISTORIES AND CASE STUDIES

Case histories (Feigenberg, 1977; Pattison, 1977; Farncombe and Chater, 1993; McLean, 1993) and case studies (Kayser-Jones and Kapp, 1989; Pearson, 1991; Bergen, 1992), have traditionally been popular in medicine and nursing (Meier and Pugh, 1986). As described by Hutchinson (1990, p.181), case histories tend to be descriptive, whereas case studies are analytical (Table 2), although case studies sometimes incorporate much of the essence of case histories in their attempts to describe, verify or generate theory.

Table 2. A comparison of case studies and case histories

	Case histories	Case studies
Topic	A life experience or an event, decision, programme, institution, organisation	A life experience or an event, decision, programme, institution, organisation
Purpose	To present the fullest possible story	To describe, verify or generate theory
Relevance of theory	Minor focus (from none to minimal)	Major focus
Style	Descriptive/narrative	Analytical/abstract

In other words, the boundaries between case histories and case studies occasionally overlap. This is well illustrated by the use of case studies in the field of death and dying. For instance, 'cases' of patients' experiences have been presented to illustrate not only the different expressions and responses of dying patients but also to support theoretical postulations about the process of dying (Pattison, 1977). Feigenberg (1977) used data from individual case histories from clinical psychiatric work with dying cancer patients to elicit 'spectra' or 'pairs of opposites' of expressions seen by health care workers. Sociologists such as Strauss and Glaser (1970) used the case history of a patient to illuminate the process of 'lingering dying' from advanced cancer. More recently, Mclean (1993), a nurse, produced vignettes of eight patients with acute leukaemia to illustrate the impact of the illness on those patients. Although these studies have incorporated interviews or participant and non-participant observations, case studies come in a variety of forms and do not preclude the use of quantitative methods (Yin, 1989).

SUMMARY

This review has highlighted some of the principal tools and methods used in studies on death and dying in health care settings. These studies have been aimed mostly at gathering data in order to provide further understanding of patients' views on dying or the behaviours of health care professionals towards them. Earlier studies used experimental designs to test behavioural and psychological differences. The use of such methods has its strengths and weaknesses. For instance, the method of controlling and analysing specified variables is more likely to produce internally valid, reliable and repeatable findings. However, such an approach invariably loses the depth and detail of complex interactions that occur between people and their environments. In contrast, use of case studies appears more relevant to studies of death and dying, which are multidimensional phenomena and, as such, maintain an interactive relationship with people, situations and environments. In case studies, multiple sources of data are collected from people, situations or environments in order to illuminate such phenomena. This method either uses interviews, participant observation or a combination of the two. The advantage is that multiple sources of data allow complex issues to be presented from a more rounded and complete perspective (Hammersley, 1992). A disadvantage is that the analysis of multiple forms of data is far from simple. For instance, contradictory findings are likely and data do not simply exist, but may have to be constructed (Ackroyd and Hughes, 1992).

It is important, therefore, when planning research into death and dying, to consider the variety of tools and methods that have been used and the advantages and disadvantages of each.

II: Exploring the experiences of patients and their nurses: methodology of the study

4. Analysing accounts of patients' experiences and those of their nurses

My analysis was conducted in three blocks of time: May-July 1992, September-December 1993 and May-July 1994. In each period of analysis the raw data were collated, coded and comparative analyses were performed. The first two blocks of analyses preceded further periods of data collection, whereas the third block followed the completion of data collection.

Carney's (1990) 'ladder of analytical abstraction' (Fig 6) was used as a guiding framework in the initial stages of the analysis. However, it became increasingly clear that the dividing line between describing and explaining data was not clear cut and did not adhere to the set boundaries as shown in this figure. Carney's (1990) framework was, nevertheless, a useful guide in planning and performing the different levels of data analysis.

The analysis and interpretation of data were conducted at two levels. The macro-level focused on gaining an overall prospective view of the phenomenon of dying and death experiences within and between cases. This involved creating a data base and writing short case summaries for each patient (see chapter 5). Notes, jottings and diagrams were integrated to build up a picture of each case. Profiles of the 12 cases were gradually built up and collated. The raw data consisted of demographic data, field observations, nursing and medical notes, tape-recorded interviews, and written notes of individual patients and their nurses.

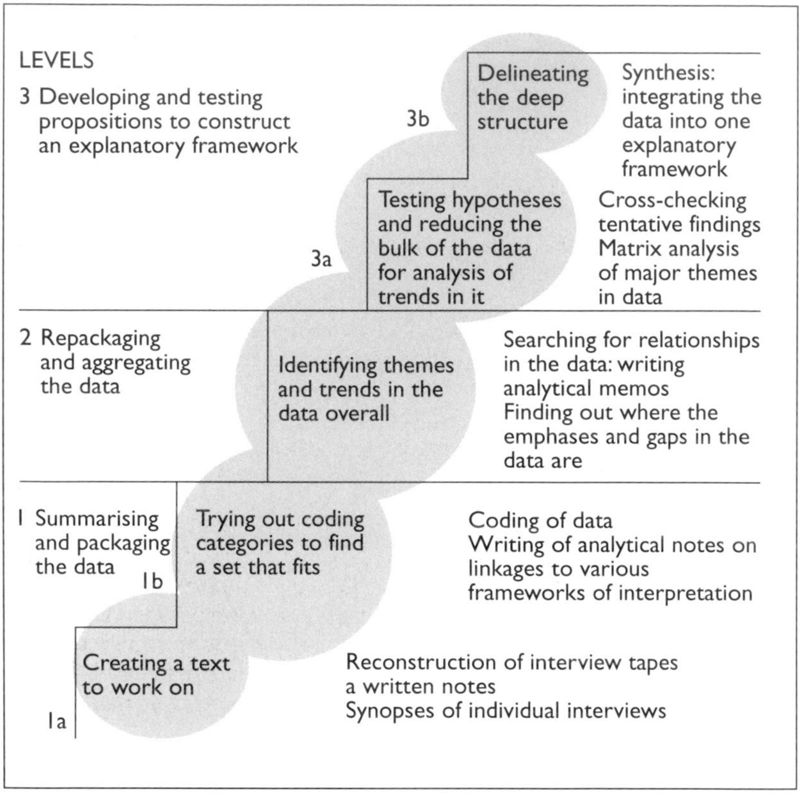

Fig 6 The ladder of analytical abstraction (after Carney, 1990)

Reprinted by permission of Sage Publications, Inc. from Carney in *Qualitative Data Analysis* by M. Miles, 1994

The tape-recorded interviews were a crucial source of data as they were a direct record of the conversations of the people concerned and therefore underpinned the whole notion of the study: to capture how individuals construe their experiences of death and dying. The tape-recordings were transcribed and analysed according to the 'grounded theory approach' (Strauss, 1987; Strauss and Corbin, 1990). This was the micro-level of analysis that aimed to assign codes and then develop and refine categories as part of the process towards developing theory. Both levels of analyses often overlapped and were at times performed in tandem with one another.

MACRO-LEVEL OF ANALYSIS: CREATING A CASE-STUDY DATA BASE

Collating evidence from multiple sources

An important part of the analysis was to explore the data in depth by looking at all the evidence for each particular case. This involved separating the material into three sets of data grouped under the headings: data arising from patients, data arising from nurses and my personal observations of the cases.

Case summaries

Case summaries of the critical events of patients' experiences and the impact of these events on the nurses were written using Weisman's (1972) method of illuminating 'critical junctures' or points of maximum interest. They subsequently formed an important aspect of the data analysis and covered three key areas — admission, medical and social history, interim events and terminal period. The summaries set out the prospective nature of the cases as they unfolded by locating the key events and the responses of patients and nurses to them. They served as a reference point for subsequent in-depth analysis of chronology of dying, as well as the cross-case comparisons and analysis.

MICRO-LEVEL OF ANALYSIS: DISCOVERING MEANINGS AND GENERATING THEORETICAL PROPOSITIONS

Immersion in the data

Initially, each transcript of recorded interview was read in conjunction with listening to the tapes. During this stage, the data were explored using Mostyn's (1985) guidelines:

- Incidence of occurrence of a particular feeling or attitude. For instance, did all the individuals express the same feeling?

- Direction and intensity of feelings expressed were explored.

- Absence or presence of a particular content. Mostyn highlighted that, according to Berelson (1971) and Gottschlack (1969), in analysing qualitative work it is equally important to bear in mind that what is *not* said may be just as important as what *is* said.

- Examination for indications of salience — that is, how willing have the people been to ensure that their actions are congruent with their stated intentions?

- Communication of individual patients and nurses — for example, people often communicate their hopes, fears and fantasies in some recognisable form so that they make sense. It is therefore crucial to ask: what does this person mean? What are they trying to say?

Notes were made on those aspects of the data that appeared to provide leads or clues for further analysis.

Coding

The second stage involved coding raw data from the transcripts (Corbin, 1986; Strauss, 1987; Miles and Huberman, 1994). Coding means creating 'tags or labels for assigning units of meaning to the descriptive or inferential information compiled during the study' (Miles and Huberman, 1994, p.56). Codes are attached to words, phrases, sentences or whole paragraphs, connected or unconnected to a specific setting but, crucially, it is not the words themselves but their meanings that are coded. Code names may take the form of a straightforward category label or a more complex one, particularly when metaphors are used.

This process followed the guidelines proposed by Strauss (1987), which have been used in several nursing studies (Melia, 1987; Field, 1989; Lawler, 1991; Smith, 1992). During the coding, the data were manually broken down sentence by sentence, in order to look for incidents and facts, and these were categorised as shown in excerpt 1 below. Several authors have cautioned against the literal equation of a word or phrase as 'meaning' (Bliss et al, 1983; Strauss, 1987; Miles and Huberman, 1994). For instance, Miles and Huberman (1994, p.56) highlighted that the meaning arising from a word or phrase occurs primarily 'by being a choice made about its significance in a given context'. Consequently, during this initial process of descriptive coding, I tried to avoid the literal equation of a word or phrase as meaning.

In order not to lose sight of the context in which the words were located, Strauss' (1987) coding paradigm, namely, 'conditions', 'interactions among actors', 'strategies and tactics' and 'consequences' was also used as a guide. These four elements enabled meanings to be uncovered by locating them in the context in which the framing and construction of situations were experienced. Strauss (1987) suggested asking the following questions: How did a particular action (or non-action) occur? Under what conditions did it occur? In what shape or form did this particular situation/phenomenon occur? What were the people saying, doing and thinking? What were the consequences for patients and nurses? Similar coding paradigms (for review see Miles and Huberman, 1994) have also been suggested by Lofland (1971) and Bogdan and Biklen (1992). The following excerpt provides an example of how the raw data were initially coded. To preserve confidentiality, all names have been changed. They are indicated by the first letter of their fictitious names whenever extracts are presented from transcripts and notes. I am GC.

Coding Excerpt 1 - Example of initial coding
Case 2 (Carol) Date: (C:15/11/91)

Transcript *Categories*

GC   You know that Susan has died, and Jane. The three of you were together for some time. How does that leave you when you see that happen?

Carol   The only thing I can think is I remember how Jane was feeling and the only thing I can feel is kind of relief really for her because she was suffering.

feeling for others and self

I know she said to me she wouldn't mind if she died.

conversations about mortality with other patients

I know the feeling. If you're not getting any better. But Susan of course was a lot younger but very sad for her. But we've all got to go sometime.

attitude to own death

Transcript		*Categories*
GC	Does that make you look at yourself when it happens?	
Carol	Yes. I often wonder how I'll go.	thoughts about own death
GC	How do you think you'll go?	
Carol	I don't know. I just hope I go in my sleep and don't know about it.	hopes to die in sleep
GC	When these thoughts go through your mind, like they do with all of us, how does that make you feel when you're thinking about death and dying?	
Carol	I guess I'm pretty fatalistic. It doesn't worry me. It doesn't really bother me.	attitude to own death
	In fact I think what use am I, as I am. I think there must be something better up there than there is here.	belief in other world
GC	Do you believe in that?	
Carol	Yes I do.	confirming belief
GC	Do you have a religion?	
Carol	Yes, I'm a Roman Catholic.	personal faith/religion
	I don't really believe in hell or anything. I think you get that here.	view of present world

Generation of categories

Once the initial coding had been performed, categories were generated according to the key themes and the information was stored in the computer. A word processing package Microsoft Word for Windows 2.0 was used. Each statement was indexed according to patient/nurse initials and transcript page numbers, as shown in excerpt 2 below.

Comparative analysis
Individual cases

The process of reading through the transcripts, listening to the tapes, coding and comparing items within individual categories by asking questions enabled the content to be analysed using a system of constant comparative analysis (Strauss 1987). During this process, diagrams, notes or memos were again made to enable themes to be pursued.

As this process continued, common patterns of dying were seen to emerge regularly and these common patterns were grouped together as a main core category. In total, 12 main categories and 40 sub-categories were generated. This process is similar to the process of 'pattern coding' (Miles and Huberman, 1994) or generating 'core categories' (Strauss 1987). This continued until no new substantive information emerged, when a particular category was judged as being saturated. Comparative analysis was, therefore, a process of comparing incident with incident and grouping summarised segments of data into a smaller number of sets, themes or constructs. Excerpt 2 below, taken from part of a patient's transcribed conversation, provides an example of how this was performed. It demonstrates the sequential process of an individual's construction of personal death and the relational aspects of this experience in comparison with the deaths of family members and other patients in similar situations.

Comparative analysis

Excerpt 2 — Example of generating core categories
Case 2 (Carol) – Segments of phrases and statements from patient transcripts

Constructing death (Core category)

Feelings for others and self (sub-category 1)

(C: 17/5/91: p.5)

Carol Just that they were out of their misery, that's the only way it affected me. Sad, but at least they weren't suffering any more.

(C: 15/11/91:p.3)

Carol   The only thing I can think is I remember how Jane was feeling and the only thing I can feel is kind of relief really for her because she was suffering. I know she said to me she wouldn't mind if she died. I know the feeling. If you're not getting any better. But Susan of course was a lot younger but very sad for her.

Attitude to death (sub-category 2)

(C: 15/11/91: p.3)

Carol   But we've all got to go sometime.

Carol   I'm not het up about it or anything.

Thoughts and wishes of own death (sub-category 3)

(C: 17/5/91: p.4)

Carol   Maybe not so much years ago. Having had my husband with me I didn't want to die, I think that's why he got me through it so many times, but I don't have a husband now. They did tell me in the United States that the next time I get cancer it will be the last time, so I've got that in my mind that this will be the last time. I can't see what they can do with a bone cancer. I think all they can do is prolong the illness and I'm not eating so I'm losing a lot of weight as well. I used to say death didn't scare me — I think it does a little because of the unknown. I think I'd rather die than live in agony.

Carol   You just take each day as it comes.

Carol   Just go peacefully.

(C: 15/11/91: p.3)

Carol   Yes. I often wonder how I'll go.

Carol   I don't know. I just hope I go in my sleep and don't know about it.

Caro   I guess I'm pretty fatalistic. It doesn't worry me. It doesn't really bother me. In fact, I think what use am I as I am. I think there must be something better up there than there is here.

Carol   I have no idea. I've seen Jane linger on so long and I wouldn't want to be in that state and last a long time. At the moment I can move around and she couldn't. So I don't know how long. I look at myself and how much weight I've lost and I think you can't lose much more.

Carol   I think so. I don't think there's a night that I go to bed that I don't think well, you know, I wonder if I'll die in my sleep. But I'm not sad about it.

Learning and observing death and dying (sub-category 4)

Watching other patients (sub-category 4: dimension 1)

(C: 17/5/91: p.5)

Carol   I've seen a few in here die too.

Carol   Just that they were out of their misery, that's the only way it affected me. Sad, but at least they weren't suffering any more.

(C: 15/11/91: p.3)

Carol   I have no idea. I've seen Jane linger on so long and I wouldn't want to be in that state and last a long time. At the moment I can move around and she couldn't. So I don't know how long. I look at myself and how much weight I've lost and I think you can't lose much more.

Watching family members (sub-category 4: dimension 2)

(C: 17.5.91)

Carol   Yes, he (referring to husband) died of cancer.

GC   Did you nurse him?

Carol   Yes, I did. His cancer was from Vietnam. He made the Agent Orange and sprayed it, and they've just acknowledged it.

Carol   I nursed him for 18 months. I nursed my mother with cancer for a few days, she didn't live very long.

Carol   My husband went into a coma and my mother had a heart attack and died in her sleep, which was a nice way to go. That's how I'd like to go.

Carol   Maybe not so much years ago. Having had my husband with me I didn't want to die, I think, that's why he got me through it so many times, but I don't have a husband now. They did tell me in the United States that the next time I get cancer it will be the last time, so I've got that in my mind that this will be the last time. I can't see what they can do with a bone cancer. I think all they can do is prolong the illness and I'm not eating so I'm losing a lot of weight as well. I used to say death didn't scare me — I think it does a little because of the unknown. I think I'd rather die than live in agony.

Death plans (sub-category 5)

Body disposal (sub-category 5: dimension 1)

(C: 17/5/91: pp.5 and 6)

Carol   He listens. I don't want to be cremated but I felt, well, I'd be cremated and have my remains sent out and buried with my husband. But now I don't know whether to or not. I think it will be a big performance for my son to do. It would be easier for him to just have me buried over here and be done with it.

Carol   As I say, I never liked cremation but my husband was cremated... I really don't know. I think I'm pretty easy about that. Whichever comes easiest for my son.

(C: 15/11/91: pp.3 and 4)

Carol   No, I don't want to be cremated, but I was going to be because my husband was cremated and I could be buried with him in the States if I wanted. But I've been thinking about not doing that because of my son. So I think I'll just be buried. Over in England.

Carol   I have done. I've shown him a few hints and that. He said well, whatever you want is what I'll do. I said I don't know what I do want.

Carol   I don't want a big ceremony. I told him: don't spend all the money on a coffin.

Carol   He takes it the same way. What he thinks deep down I don't know. But... he takes it the same way. He doesn't dwell on it or anything.

Carol   I think so at the moment, than send me out there. He's got all the work to do to arrange it all. So I think it would be easier to be buried over here.

GC   But would you in your heart of hearts like to be with Alan?

Carol   Yes, if I could. Without causing a lot of trouble.

Material disposal (sub-category 5: dimension 2)

(C: 17/5/91: pp.6)

Carol   Not really. Kind of but not as much as I would have liked. My son is going to have an awful lot of rummaging through papers, but I do have a will.

Cross-case comparisons and 'conceptual mapping'

The process of comparative analysis was repeated for every patient and nurse transcript, then the relationships between individual patients' and nurses' core categories and sub-categories were collated and explored as a whole. Often this involved drawing diagrams, analysing background data, tracking down conditions and relationships between categories and asking questions using Strauss' (1987) coding paradigm. An example of this conceptual mapping showing the interplay between nurse-patient are shown in Figs 7 and 8 respectively.

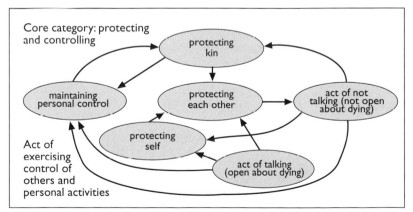

Fig 7 Conceptual mapping and diagramming

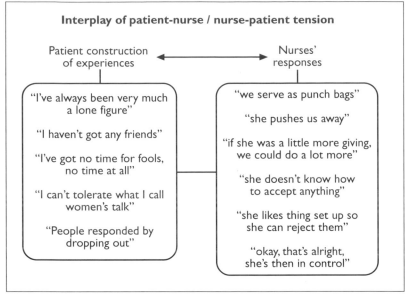

Interplay of patient-nurse / nurse-patient tension

Patient construction of experiences ⟷ Nurses' responses

"I've always been very much a lone figure"

"I haven't got any friends"

"I've got no time for fools, no time at all"

"I can't tolerate what I call women's talk"

"People responded by dropping out"

"we serve as punch bags"

"she pushes us away"

"if she was a little more giving, we could do a lot more"

"she doesn't know how to accept anything"

"she likes thing set up so she can reject them"

"okay, that's alright, she's then in control"

Fig 8 Display of patient-nurse/nurse-patient construction of situation, as seen in case 8

Eventually, this process of conceptual mapping involved a period of selective coding (Strauss, 1987). A decision had to be made with regard to which categories were central to the present research. This part of the analysis was useful for explicating a 'story line' and integrating the central categories. According to Strauss and Corbin (1990), laying down a story line involves moving from description to conceptualisation. It involves making hard choices between two or more salient phenomena, particularly if tight, dense integration and development of the categories are to be achieved. Hence, an important part of this particular phase of the analysis was to return to the original research questions.

This provided an anchor for testing out which aspects of the data were most central to the research. Finally, the categories were subsumed into three main core themes: the 'acts of protecting and controlling', the 'acts of watching and waiting' and the 'acts of holding on and letting go'. These were given titles based on metaphors, used by the patients themselves to express their experiences (see Chapter 5). These metaphors captured first hand both the sequential patterns and reality of individuals' experiences during the process of dying.

CROSS-CHECKING THE INTERPRETATION OF MEANINGS DURING ANALYSIS

This was conducted at several levels.

During data collection

My own interpretation of situations and events was subjected to cross-checking for reliability to increase the credibility of the analysis. During data collection, information and meanings obtained from the previous interview were checked with the participants for consistency before the follow-up interview began, and at its end. Nursing and medical notes, and the observations of nurses and medical staff, were used as additional checks.

During coding

A modified system of external review of the coding process was used. A sample of three sets of data was independently coded by two colleagues who had previous experience of coding data of this type. Their coding was compared for consistency with my own, and considerable levels of agreement were observed. Derivation of evidence and interpretations of the transcripts were also scrutinised, followed by questions for clarification. This helped establish consistency and gave me additional confidence in the system of coding.

During comparative analyses

A process of cross-referencing of codes and evidence, within and between cases, was used to increase confidence in the findings. The relationships between core categories were outlined and supporting events or incidents traced. This tracing of conditional paths enabled conditions and consequences to be directly linked with action/interaction (Strauss and Corbin, 1990). For example, the pattern of 'protecting', as constructed by the dying person, can be traced to three main acts: protecting kin, protecting nurse and protecting self. The application of these cross-checks — checking for researcher effects on the case and vice versa, using multiple sources of data and weighing of evidence — helped introduce elementary safeguards.

5. Case summaries

Death and dying form a distinctive part of a life history. It is difficult to imagine our dying and death as being the same as another person's because, ultimately, no two individuals are alike in every way. Nevertheless, there are elements of dying that appear to be commonly experienced. Therefore, when considering death and dying as a phenomenon it is important to take into account both the individual and the common aspects of the experience.

Furthermore, the decision to enter a hospice as a patient is a symbolic one. The act is a defining process and may signal a number of meanings to the patient, relatives and professional carers. For instance, for the patient it may mean that medical cure is less likely, if not impossible. Instead, the prime focus for the rest of that person's life will be centred on care and the management of pain and symptoms in the hope of achieving a reasonable quality of life. For the patients in this study, entering a hospice marked a phase of their lives where personal meanings of living and dying, values and goals in life were likely to become central issues of increasing daily concern. For the nurses, too, it represented an equally critical juncture. The initial meeting with the patient provided an opportunity to demonstrate humane care, concern and respect. This patient-nurse/nurse-patient encounter sets the scene for the subsequent social construction of both in defining the nature of expectations, delivery and reception of care.

The names of all concerned in the study have been changed to protect confidentiality. The years showing the period of care and treatments have been purposely omitted. The months have been retained to maintain the timing of events as they occurred.

Case summary 1: Susan

Age: 46

Period of contact: *Six months*

Number of conversations with Susan: *Six*

Number of conversations with her nurses: *Five*

Place of death: *Hospice*

Admission, medical and social history

Susan was 46 years old and grew up in Cheshire. She was married to James, a headmaster. They had three children, Tom, 14, and Jane and Tony, in their early 20s. Susan presented with a three-year history of metastatic carcinoma of the breast with bony secondaries. She underwent a left mastectomy and was referred at her request to the hospice in December, for relaxation and support and subsequently for pain and symptom control as her cancer rapidly progressed. Her bone scan showed widespread deposits in her sacro-iliac joints and right humerus.

Susan talked freely to her nurses about her illness and her dying. She was often sad and tearful when talking about her own losses, particularly in not being able to be part of her children's future. Susan's own childhood was a lonely one. She said that her parents were not warm people and, although they cared for her materially, in Susan's words they were not particularly loving. Consequently, Susan was determined to bring up her children in a family unit with love and warmth. At the time of the study, Susan's mother had died. Her 82-year-old father was alive. Susan had always attended church regularly and her faith was significant to her.

Interim events

Following her referral, Susan participated in the activities of the day centre, such as massage and relaxation, which she enjoyed. She was mobile and able to drive herself to and from home but found it increasingly tiring if she exerted herself. At the same time she appeared to derive benefit from her course of steroid therapy, pamidronate treatment and radiotherapy.

Susan's nurses described her as someone who was anxious. She was open about her illness and able to be talk about it. The most profound impact of Susan's experience on her nurses was her grief and sorrow at her imminent mortality. This ranged from tangible, physical losses to more philosophical and searching elements of loss such as her own mortality and, alongside that, a deep sense of spiritual pain. As Susan put it: 'I just think: we've been married 25 years this year. I don't know what I've done to deserve it, really. I know it's silly looking at it now... but I've never smoked, never drink alcohol... only occasionally. I've just led a very simple life... you just think, why?'

Seven months after her referral, in July, Susan fell at home and became extremely anxious, perceiving the fall as a sign that her disease was spreading. She had also become more breathless and was particularly concerned that this change in her body would not affect her holiday with her husband and Tom, their youngest child. Tom and Susan had drawn up a list of things to do, and the holiday was included. Susan's condition did not deteriorate any further and she was able to go on holiday in August which the whole family enjoyed.

On her return, Susan's condition deteriorated rapidly. Her cancer had spread to her liver and there were further metastases in her bones, with spinal cord compression. Susan was given blood transfusions to help increase her haemoglobin and platelet levels and to alleviate her breathlessness. According to Susan's nurse, James and Susan for the first time came to see her as a couple to talk about their anxieties. As her nurse put it: 'Because they've been a close couple they haven't really been able to share the illness together. They have been contending with it separately. They are close, but they can't share because they have been trying to protect each other.' James talked openly about his anxieties and conflicts of duties — wanting to care for Susan at home and having to work. Susan listened and was able to do that without looking upset. The impression of the nurse was that 'a whole series has happened quite dramatically and Susan is less fearful... although things are deteriorating, she is accepting more and isn't as fearful...'

Terminal period

During September, Susan continued to attend the day centre and was admitted for short periods of time for blood transfusions and investigations as she continued to deteriorate. She found it difficult to come to terms with her situation and wanted to keep going for as long as she could. As Susan said: 'I'm going to try and keep going as long as I can. I am not going to give up. Even if they can give me a blood transfusion every month to keep me going... I'm quite happy to do that.' She also expressed her desire to die in the hospice and not at home.

Susan was subsequently admitted to the ward via the day centre. She was breathless and experiencing severe back pain. She appeared very low. A nursing entry read: 'Quiet, not talking, like Susan normally enjoys. Had spoken to another patient about her fear of dying; feeling as though she was being trapped by her body which was not letting her die. She just wants to be taken from this situation.' During the next five days Susan remained breathless, despite further blood transfusions, and was in considerable mental anguish. She was aware of her deterioration and was frightened and expressed the desire to die asleep and peacefully. She made plans for her funeral arrangements. Susan was determined to continue with further interventions, such as blood transfusions and an epidural, to relieve her back pain. The latter was cancelled because of her low platelet count. On the fifth day following her admission, Susan requested sedation so she could sleep and be calmer. Her family were informed of her rapidly deteriorating condition and were at her bedside. She asked her husband and family if it was all right for her to 'let go'. Her family gave her permission to do so. Susan continued to deteriorate that afternoon, became unconscious with noisy breathing and, before her death, leaked faecal discharge from her mouth. She died the following morning. Her death was described by her nurse as 'difficult' and distressing for her, her family and the nurses.

Case summary 2: Carol

Age: *60*

Period of contact: *14 months*

Number of conversations with Carol: *12*

Number of conversations with her nurses: *10*

Place of death: *Hospice*

Admission, medical and social history

Carol was of Irish descent, born in London, the only child from her mother's second marriage. Both her half-sister and brother were much older and Carol grew up effectively as an only child. Her father died from cancer when she was 10. Her mother had died many years before from cancer of the oesophagus.

Carol presented with a 17-year-history of breast cancer. She had had bilateral mastectomies and presented with bony secondaries in July. Until then, her disease was stable and slow in progress. Carol married her first husband at 17 and had a 42-year-old son, Mike. Before marriage she was a professional ballroom dancer and a child prodigy, travelling all over the country, doing shows for the troops during the war years. Her first marriage ended in divorce and some years later Carol married Alan, an American ex-serviceman, whom she adored. She went to live in the USA. Mike, her son, remained with his father. Her life in the United States was happy until Carol was diagnosed with breast cancer. Alan was her source of support, particularly when her cancer was diagnosed. Each time she had a setback with her disease, Carol said that it was always Alan who had got her through. However, he was then also diagnosed with cancer and died in the early 1970s. His cancer was attributed to the use of Agent Orange in Vietnam. Carol had always felt that her husband would survive her, and his illness and death were therefore significant. Carol returned to live in England. She subsequently found that her cancer had spread to her bones.

Apart from her son Mike, her dog, visits from her priest and her friend, Dorothy, Carol appeared to live a rather lonely life, on her own in a council bungalow. She had no close family contacts and ties. Carol described herself as 'not overly religious' but, at the same time, believed in her Roman Catholicism, and her faith was important to her.

Interim events

Carol was referred by her GP in November for pain and symptom control. She was admitted as a day-centre patient and participated in the social activities held there. Throughout her time in the hospice Carol was always immaculate in her personal grooming. According to her nurses she was the only patient on the ward who 'wore silk pyjamas and looked glamorous right until the last few days before her death'. Although Carol was perceived by staff as a woman with immaculate social graces, she was also described by them as a private person. At times, her nurse reported that she was content not to converse or, if she did, to talk about superficial issues. Physically, Carol was mobile and looked well. She was on a course of pamidronate, which alleviated much of the pain she was experiencing from secondaries in her bones.

Carol remained in a fairly stable physical condition for the next eight months. She was admitted to the ward for short periods for reassessment and treatment of her pain and was discharged when she improved. During that year there were no significant physical changes in Carol's condition.

During this time I was able to get to know Carol rather better. She was happy to talk to me and, although not forthcoming in depth, often the issues she raised were pertinent. She talked openly about her dying, declaring that she was 'pretty fatalistic' about it. Carol continued: 'It doesn't worry me. It doesn't really bother me. In fact, I think: what use am I as I am? I think there must be something better up there then there is here... yes, I'm a Roman Catholic... I don't really believe in hell or anything. I think you get that here.'

Carol appeared quite philosophical about her situation and told me that when her husband was alive she did not want to die. However, she felt that this was the 'last time', and, apart from prolonging her illness, she could not see what 'they (the doctors) can do with bone cancer'.

Two years after her admission, in early March, concerns were expressed by her Macmillan nurse who noticed a significant change in Carol, albeit a gradual one. She said that Carol was deteriorating and, although opportunities had been created to talk about her change in condition, Carol's conversation with her remained superficial. I visited Carol at her home together with her Macmillan nurse. Carol looked pale and was in bed in a small bedroom. She was unable to read, as she could not find the energy to do so, but enjoyed listening to songs from her radio. Her dog was with her. She was pleased to see us and the conversation centred around physical aspects of her care. Carol was experiencing pain and her medication was reviewed. This was subsequently followed up by the Macmillan nurse with Carol's GP.

Terminal period

The following month, Carol was admitted to the ward. She had deteriorated and was feeling nauseated. She had lost a considerable amount of weight but, despite feeling unwell, her attention to her physical appearance remained immaculate. This admission was important because it raised several issues for the team of nurses on the ward. Nursing Carol appeared difficult — in part a consequence of Carol's lack of openness about how she was really feeling. This created considerable soul-searching among the nurses who believed that their offers of help and support were rejected by Carol. The interviews with the nurses revealed feelings of helplessness. During this admission Carol appeared more and more withdrawn. The nurses found her withdrawal and lack of reciprocity difficult to comprehend and, therefore, had difficulty making progress with her care. Throughout her illness Carol maintained a calm, accepting, albeit ambivalent attitude towards her death, which was never explicitly expressed. This became increasingly prominent when talk of being discharged home was put to her by the medical team. Some of the nurses felt that Carol would not be able to cope, but she chose to go home. The tension created here was due in part to not really knowing what was in Carol's mind.

Carol was readmitted at her own request after a fortnight at home. During this admission she was brighter and talked about preparations for her funeral and how she had talked to her son about not buying an expensive coffin.

Two weeks after this admission Carol requested to go home. By this time she was physically fading away. She appeared to have lost more weight and looked increasingly frail. She continued attendance at the day centre until the middle of June. Carol fell at home and fractured the odontoid peg of her cervical vertebra. On admission she was in considerable pain and could only lie flat on her back. She continued to deteriorate and died a week later 'without struggle' in an unconscious state. Her son was not present at her death but visited later. Throughout Carol's illness he had found the whole process 'difficult'.

Case summary 3: Jane

Age: *60*

Period of contact: *Seven months*

Number of conversations with Jane: *Six*

Number of conversations with her nurses: *Five*

Place of death: *Home*

Admission, medical and social history

Jane was born and raised in east London and used to work in a home for delinquent children. She was married to Ron and they had two grown-up children, Joy and Joseph. Jane was 60 years old and was described by her nurses as 'articulate, witty, a natural conversationalist', who talked openly about her disease and dying in a matter-of-fact way. She grew up in wartime London with her brother, who was killed in the war. Jane said that she had had a rich childhood despite hard times. After their marriage, Ron and Jane moved out of London and lived in a village in the country. Her father died about eight years earlier, leaving Jane's 88-year-old mother, who lived in London. Jane was an 'atheist', although she was brought up as 'Church of England'.

Jane was first referred in February for pain and symptom control. She was diagnosed to have disseminated carcinoma of the breast with bony secondaries. Her bone scan showed widespread deposits throughout the skeleton. At the time of referral Jane was mobile, but in general her mobility was greatly hampered by the extent of her disease. She was in constant pain and, although medication helped take the edge off her pain in the months that followed, Jane continued to live with a niggling pain, which she bore with great fortitude.

Interim events

During the next 12 months, Jane attended the day centre and appeared to make a tremendous impression on patients and staff. A large part of this was due to her personality, which was larger than life. She drew people into her company, participated and contributed to the activities of the day centre and supported both patients and staff. She was described as 'much loved by all the staff' and as someone with 'a real charismatic personality'. During this period Jane underwent further chemotherapy and pamidronate treatment and overall was able to maintain much of her independence. Her greatest fear, which she expressed openly, was becoming incontinent.

In March, Jane's physical deterioration became more marked. This was a significant event. Jane was admitted. She could only lie on her back and was unable to move as her cancer had progressed extensively to her spine. She was in tremendous pain. She talked about her cancer and dying openly to me and to the nurses who cared for her. Often, when I talked to her, she would use humour. An entry in her nursing notes read: 'Jane talked about her cancer. Said she should have been dead months ago. She feels she has accepted her illness. Has no regrets. Has had a good life and 60 happy years. Said that knowing that she is going to die has meant that she is able to put her affairs in order. She feels that her quality of life at present is reasonable, despite being bedfast — she can still read and have a laugh. Her main fear is of becoming doubly incontinent or paralysed. She feels she could not cope with loss of her dignity.'

Paradoxically, Jane's openness and 'being brave' about her condition appeared to make some of the nurses caring for her uneasy. Most of her nurses thought her apparent bravery was a 'front', in part because she wanted to remain strong and was consequently having to project this image all the time. There was a feeling that Jane was not really as brave as she appeared and there was a very private side to her, despite her apparent openness. Some nurses found it difficult to broach this subject with her.

In June I visited Jane at her home, together with the Macmillan nurse. This was primarily to assess her slurred speech and drowsiness. Jane thought this was due to her deteriorating condition and was disappointed when it was thought that it was more likely due to the side effects of metoclopromide, a drug to control feelings of nausea and vomiting, because according to her, she was 'ready to go'. Her husband was very welcoming and took the opportunity of our presence to take the dog for a walk. Jane was alert and chatty and, although pale, she still managed to put her lipstick on. She said how tired she had been of living and talked about the merits of euthanasia. She was not worried about dying but rather how she was going to die.

By July there was evidence of further spinal cord compression, and Jane was barely able to move her legs at all. Her pain was worse and she was admitted for further assessment and respite. She lay flat on her back and often would talk to me about how it made her look at the world from a different viewpoint.

Jane continued to deteriorate steadily and during this admission her bladder and bowel control began to deteriorate. She was leaking urine and the nurse looking after her said that she found any procedure connected with continence 'painful and degrading'. The nurses were therefore particularly sensitive in dealing with her lack of bladder control. Discussions occurred between Jane and the nurses about how best to help her with this. Medical examination confirmed that she had developed urinary retention.

Catheterisation was suggested, but Jane was deeply upset and said that this was the 'last straw'. She expressed the desire to die. Meanwhile, attempts were made, using conservative measures such as regular toileting, to see if Jane could empty her bladder. She and her nurses continued for 24 hours but gradually Jane acknowledged that she would end up with an infection if she continued to leak urine. She was catheterised the next day with her consent. Her relief was instant and she said that she could not believe why she had not had a catheter before.

Jane remained on the ward for a further four days. Her spirits were considerably dampened and she became withdrawn and low in mood. Her bone pains were difficult to alleviate and Jane declined the offer of an epidural. She wanted to go home. Jane was discharged home with a package of ongoing support and care during the last week of July.

Terminal period

At home Jane deteriorated slowly and remained confined to bed. She was nursed by her husband, supported by the community and Macmillan nursing team. In mid-October I visited for the final time. During this visit Jane talked about her death and how she hoped that when it happened it would be fairly quick. She said that she had long passed her time and expected to live only for another two weeks.

Jane died quietly, without struggle, on a Saturday afternoon as she predicted, two weeks after our conversation. Her husband had washed and made her comfortable and she had spoken to her mother in London that morning. Her son had also visited the day before. Ron made Jane a milky drink, which she drank. He went to the kitchen to make himself a sandwich and when he returned, 20 minutes later, he found that Jane had died. Ron was sad, but composed, as he had been throughout Jane's illness.

Case summary 4: Ian

Age: *50*

Period of contact: *38 months*

Number of conversations with Ian: *15*

Number of conversations with his nurses: *16*

Living

Admission, medical and social history

Ian was born in Scotland. He had a brother, Donald, who was five years older than him and a sister who died when she was five. Ian described his childhood as a happy one, despite having been unwell between the ages of three and seven with a bout of childhood illnesses. His brother was the healthy child and, although they were not close as children, their relationship changed when they reached their late teens. Ian married at 19 but was divorced by the age of 21. He described his mother as a 'protective woman' who wanted to run his life and his father as the opposite, a man who felt he should run his own affairs.

After his divorce Ian left Scotland for London. He remarried and his relationship with his brother deepened. They kept in touch and visited each other. Donald had a stroke and became an invalid until his death from a heart attack. As Ian put it: 'He was the one that all through my life had never been ill. He'd had colds and things like that but never anything serious. Then he was hit by this. I always looked on him as the strength for the two of us and he always seemed to go through life with no... sort of setbacks... It shook me quite a lot...' During this time Ian's father died suddenly from a heart attack, leaving his mother. who subsequently became ill and, despite not wanting to move away from Scotland, she was left with no choice but to move to England to live with Ian. She too died a few years earlier.

Ian's family currently comprised his wife Pat and their two children, Sally and Trevor. Sally was married, lived locally and visited regularly.

Ian was diagnosed as having testicular teratoma at the age of 45 and underwent right orchidectomy and chemotherapy. His illness was upsetting for Donald, bringing both of them closer still. Three years after the initial treatment metastases were discovered in Ian's lungs, which were subsequently treated with another dose of chemotherapy, followed by a left lobectomy. In June he presented with a solitary lung metastasis which was excised. His condition stabilised after this recurrence and, according to his physician, his disease was thought to be in remission but it remained uncertain whether the cancer would recur.

Ian also had angina, a hiatus hernia and a long-standing history of low back pain, which had resulted in three laminectomies. He was referred to the hospice by his GP a year later for social support and pain and symptom control.

Ian was tall, well dressed, with grey hair. He wore double hearing aids, walked with the assistance of two sticks and used a wheelchair for longer journeys. He talked easily and openly and told me that, although he was a worrier, death did not frighten him: 'It never has to the degree that I would sit down and worry about it and make my illness worse. Just by worrying about that you could die.' Ian said this view had much to do with his faith. He described himself as not a 'great Christian by any means', but he had been brought up to go to church and found that his faith had helped him throughout his illness.

Interim events

Although initially apprehensive about being referred to a hospice, after a few visits Ian settled down and attended the day centre twice a week. He had an annual check-up and on such occasions he learnt to cope with the possibility of bad news by being prepared for the worst. Ian said that he faced each visit with uncertainty about future prognosis and, moreover, throughout the past five years had had to live daily with chronic pain and symptoms from his other medical problems. Often his doctors were unable to find the cause for their manifestations.

Throughout Ian's time as a day-centre patient it had been common knowledge, and a constant frustration to the nurses, that both medical and nursing staff were unable to get to grips with the multifaceted nature of his illness. As soon as a particular symptom subsided a new one would crop up. Ian constantly tried different treatment regimes and lived in a state of chronic illness. He talked openly and gave vivid accounts of his constant worries and anger. He described the 'stigma' of having to use a wheelchair outside his home and gave accounts of the loss of self-identity as a result of how people related to him — as someone with an incurable illness and as a 'cripple' and a non-person when he was in his wheelchair.

In October, following his annual check-up, it was finally confirmed by Ian's oncologist that his cancer remission was likely to be long term and that it was probable that Ian had been 'cured', although his other medical conditions remained problematic. This posed the question to the medical and nursing team of the nature of Ian's long-term care. For instance, as his nurse said, Ian's social company in the day centre was made up of patients who were dying. During the previous 18 months Ian's nurses observed that he tended not to mix socially and increasingly kept himself apart from other patients. When I talked to him about the effects the death of the other patients had on him, Ian responded that he felt sad each time but had learnt to cope with it by being more detached.

His recent medical prognosis appeared to have a profound impact on the nurses. Ian's dying trajectory was perceived as falling further outside the boundaries of someone facing impending death. Moreover, when Ian's doctor proposed discharging him from the day centre, feelings of tension, guilt, and unease were experienced and expressed by some of the nurses. Issues such as the extent to which Ian had been socialised into being 'medicalised' and adopting a 'dying role' were raised. Ian's wife had also become dependent on the facilities offered by the hospice during the previous five years, as they had given her space and time for herself. Consequently, this change would also have an impact on her and the family.

This phase of unease was tempered weeks later by a proposal that, even if Ian was to be discharged, links would still be maintained with him through out-patients, and he would still have the option of using the day centre facilities. Meanwhile, attendance at a young disabled unit was proposed as part of a transitional process of rehabilitating Ian back into living and integrating with people who were not dying. This plan was put to Ian who was, on the whole, receptive, although he did not commit himself to the idea entirely. To date, Ian's physical condition appears stabilised and he continues to be treated for his ongoing chronic physical problems. According to Ian, his remission had given him greater confidence to plan for his future. His attendance at the day centre has been reduced to once a week.

Case summary 5: Lyn

Age: *44*

Period of contact: *18 months*

Number of conversations with Lyn: *12*

Number of conversations with her nurses: *10*

Place of death: *Hospice*

Admission, medical and social history

Lyn was 44 years old. She was born in the north of England and lived there until she was seven. Much of her childhood was spent with her grandmother and godmother, and she spent very little time with her own parents, unlike her older sister who lived with her parents in their caravan, where there was not enough room for. Consequently, her relationship with her parents had never been a close one, despite living with them again from the age of seven when they moved south. Lyn said that she was closer to her work mates than to her parents and felt she 'could never discuss anything with them'.

Lyn married at 22 but later divorced, shortly after she developed breast cancer. She was working as a book-binder by then and was left to raise her two sons, Bill, aged 10, and Nick, who was only seven at the time of her diagnosis. Bill became 'delinquent' and left home in his teens, ending up serving a custodial sentence in a remand centre. Lyn's relationship with her younger son became closer, but she said she felt a sense of failure in terms of her relationship with her older son, who had become angry and openly violent to her.

By this time Lyn had developed a relationship with Paul, who was supportive, unlike her 'uncaring' ex-husband. Lyn described herself as not having any set religion. 'I know about different religions and all sorts of religions and I think they've all got their good and bad. It's up to the individual, but I've got no set religion. Once I'm gone, I'm gone,' she said.

Lyn's breast cancer was treated surgically with a segmental mastectomy, followed by chemotherapy. Her disease remained in remission for 10 years, when it was discovered that there were metastases in her bones, lungs and liver. Her oncologist referred her to the hospice for palliative care.

Lyn was a chatty person who talked openly about her condition, laughed a lot and saw the funny side of things. She was described by the nurses as having a strong personality and being a 'fighter' and overall had adopted a positive attitude towards her disease. She cycled to the day centre regularly and, although a few nurses found her cheerful front difficult to comprehend, Lyn appeared popular with the staff and patients.

Interim events

Throughout the following months, Lyn participated and contributed to the activities of the day centre. She developed friendships with the other patients and it was not unusual to find her initiating various activities that involved them. Her symptoms remained well controlled and Lyn said that her quality of life was good. She talked openly about her disease with me and her thoughts about death and dying. She had made plans to visit her godmother and aunt to talk to them about her condition. She subsequently went to see them and found the visit poignant. At the same time she had also started making plans for her funeral and was exploring the possibility of a cremation, followed by a burial of her ashes. Lyn was most concerned that Nick should have a place to go and place flowers on her grave if he wanted to. Her relationship with Bill remained estranged, and Lyn feared that he might act violently towards Nick after she died. She also tried to talk to her sister about her illness but told me that it was difficult to do so, as her sister found it upsetting. She maintained contact with her elderly parents but, because of their past history and increasing age, they were unable to provide much support.

Although many things about her family affairs remained unresolved, Lyn remained physically stable until a year later in April, when on arrival at the day centre, the nurses found that she was breathless and looked unwell. Her nurse said that although Lyn had a big smile on her face she was upset and it was the nearest they had seen her to tears. According to her nurse, Lyn was 'very frightened and worried about what was happening although she was still smiling'. She was admitted to the acute hospital, having developed pericardial effusion. She remained in hospital for three days following drainage of fluids from her chest. This episode appeared to be significant for Lyn. According to her, it indicated that her disease was progressing further. On discharge from the hospital she experienced a panic attack at home which she attributed in part to being discharged from hospital too soon, and not taking it easy, because she had attended a wedding as well as a cabaret on the weekend after her discharge.

A month later, Lyn recovered and was back to her old self. She described herself as feeling on top of the world. She had been prescribed steroids and was benefiting from their use. When asked about their effects, Lyn said: 'They do make you feel an awful lot better, because two months ago I really felt like I was going downhill… I was going downhill so fast that I didn't think I was living a lot longer.' Following further chemotherapy, Lyn continued in a fairly stable condition for another six months. This period was interrupted with the occasional episodes of breathlessness, headaches and a couple of panic attacks.

In early November the following year, Lyn's headaches and breathlessness became worse and she was admitted for assessment of pleural and pericardial disease. The CT scan showed no signs of further metastases and Lyn was assured by the doctors that her headaches were not due to any sinister cause. Diuretics were helping her and Lyn felt that she no longer wanted to pursue further treatment, although she still wanted to maintain her links with the oncologists as well as getting support from the hospice. By mid-December, Lyn's condition had deteriorated further and there were more reports of breathlessness and feelings of anxiousness.

A month later Lyn came to the day centre and appeared very ill. She looked grey, pale, felt nauseated and was coughing as well as being breathless. She had stopped taking her steroids by this time. When Lyn saw me she said: 'It's my liver! I shall be glad for a rest.' Lyn was admitted to the in-patient ward that day for symptom control with a view to being discharged home if she improved.

Terminal period

Lyn's admission lasted for four weeks until her death in early February. During this time attempts were made to alleviate her breathlessness, nausea and vomiting. She was self-caring for most of the time, requiring nursing assistance only towards the last few days of her life. She spent most of this time putting her affairs in order, particularly for Nick. Bill visited, but these visits were not particularly welcomed by Lyn, who remained unable to reconcile with her estranged older son. On such occasions the nurses, who were caught in the middle, said that they found it very difficult emotionally. On the other hand, Lyn made every effort to talk openly about her feelings and to prepare both Paul, her boyfriend, and Nick for her death. She expressed relief when this happened and the three of them were able to talk openly about how both Nick and Paul were going to cope after her death.

Lyn became increasingly tired and less steady on her feet but continued to maintain a brave front, despite her condition. On one of my visits to the ward she told me that one of the patients, whom she knew, had died in the side ward and that it had been very reassuring for her to see this person in death, as she had never seen a dead person before. This helped her to think of what it might be like for her when it happened.

However, Lyn also felt afraid that she would die too suddenly, in case it upset her son. She said that she wanted to be buried and not cremated. Her greatest fear was not death in itself but the thought that she might 'try to hang on for too long'.

The last two weeks before her death were disturbing for Lyn. She was unable to sleep and the nights were frightening for her. Often she would sleep in a reclining chair in the sitting room in the company of the night nurses. She deteriorated further and became drowsy, disorientated at times and more unsteady on her feet. Lyn declined the offer of sedation to help her with sleeping during the day. An entry in her nursing notes read: 'She still appears to want to be in control and fight her deterioration.' Her breathlessness became more acute at times and Lyn had a 'haunted' look about her. The nurse looking after her explained this phenomenon succinctly: 'The only way I could describe the weeks leading up to that [her death] was like a wounded animal who was just desperately trying to get up all the time and just couldn't rest and couldn't be at peace. She was just fighting, fighting...'

Eventually, Lyn decided that she had had enough and requested sedation to help her sleep. This decision was finally taken after a horrific nightmare in which Lyn felt that she was cut open by the surgeons and there was blood running everywhere. She woke up and the impact of the dream was so vivid that she was still wanting to be washed clean of the blood hours afterwards. This experience was traumatic both for her and the nurses. Lyn requested sedation that would enable her to have a 'deep long sleep' and not one where she would 'drift on and off'.

Both her doctor and her nurse saw Lyn and her family to negotiate how the sedation would be administered and how the consequences would impact on her current deterioration. Her family agreed with Lyn's request, after some mixed response, and Lyn was able to sleep solidly for four hours, waking up fresh. With further sedation she slept solidly throughout the night. This regime continued for three days and during this time Lyn gradually became unconscious. She died in the presence of her parents, her boyfriend Paul and her two sons. At the moment of her death Bill was distraught and shook Lyn violently, not wanting to let her go, at the same time hitting out at Paul. Although the situation eventually resolved peacefully, Lyn's last days appeared emotionally distressing for her, her family and the nurses.

Case summary 6: Alison

Age: *35*

Period of contact: *20 months*

Number of conversations with Alison: *15*

Number of conversations with her nurses: *10*

Place of death: *Hospice*

Admission, medical and social history

Alison was 35 years old and single. She was born and brought up in the north of England. She grew up in the countryside and, until the age of 14, 'did not have a care in the world'. She had a brother, Phillip, and described their relationship as follows: 'As children we fought all the time as children do, as adolescents we fought a lot. Then there's like…20…we had a great time together, and now he's married, I only see him at home.' In her teens Alison wanted to leave school early to 'travel, travel, travel', but her parents insisted that she went to catering college. She completed her course and almost immediately went off all over the world, living life to the full, with a group of girlfriends. Alison had recently started on a course in nursing as a mature student and was living in a house she jointly owned with a friend. Since leaving home she had always led an independent life.

The first indication of her illness occurred when Alison felt increasingly tired, developed 'hallucinations' and went to see her doctor. Subsequent investigations revealed that she had glioma. When the diagnosis was conveyed to her, Alison met it with disbelief, shock and responded by avoiding the use of the word 'cancer'. She preferred to use the term 'tumour'. Subsequent biopsy showed that the glioma was inoperable, and Alison began a series of treatments with chemotherapy and medication. During this time Alison's father died, which had a profound impact on her and her family. Alison was also beginning to find it 'difficult' at home. Her housemates were unable to adjust to her situation and had changed in their attitude towards her. Two years from her initial diagnosis, in September, Alison was referred for palliative care and social support.

When I first met Alison she appeared friendly and was keen to help with the research. She had been attending the day centre and took an interest in the activities offered there. According to her nurse, she enjoyed massage therapy, participated in the patient support group and was about to embark on music therapy. She was observed to make a great effort in talking to the male patients and would include them in the things she was doing. Alison's nurse described her as 'somebody who was fiercely independent, in need of control, and with a stubborn side to her underneath an easy-going and giving nature'. Her circumstances and age appeared to evoke a tremendous sense of pity and protectiveness towards her from both the staff and other patients. Alison described herself as being brought up as a Catholic and, although not initially obvious, during the latter part of her illness her faith became increasingly important to her.

Interim events

In the following months Alison remained physically stable, despite ongoing chemotherapy, radiotherapy, steroid and anticonvulsive treatments. The latter were prescribed as she had started to develop seizures. Much to Alison's distress, she had increasingly put on weight because of the steroids. Her energy was low and, as Alison put it: 'I'm slowly, sort of…like doing jobs within the house, but it takes me a long time and I accept it now that it takes a long time… yesterday, it took me all day to cut the grass, which usually takes a couple of hours…' This period of 'plateauing' with peaks and troughs appeared as the main features of Alison's disease progression.

According to her nurse, in between Alison's physical treatments much of her care involved working with her at an emotional level. Alison implied that she was aware that the prognosis of her cancer was poor and often said to her nurse that she found each setback, in the form of new symptoms, hard to accept. She was often tearful and talked about her losses openly, particularly to her nurse at the day centre, whom she trusted. Her grief about her multiple losses and impending death appeared very deep and raw. As Alison put it: 'I think each day you think about it. Some days I think: yes, okay, I'll accept it, and other days I'll cry, thinking: why me? and going through all those stages again.' Throughout the following months Alison continued to live with uncertainty, hope and progressive losses.

In January the following year, Alison's seizures returned, this time more frequent. She looked unwell and appeared to be lacking in energy and afraid of going out on her own. Her medications were reassessed and slowly, in the weeks that followed, Alison appeared better. By April, her home situation with her housemates had worsened and they requested that Alison should move out. This further rejection was hurtful and distressing for her. She moved to a self-contained flat and, despite her unsteadiness, maintained her independence and went on a summer holiday to the USA, on her own, to visit her relatives. Alison came back from her trip full of excitement at her achievement.

By September, Alison's nurse reported that there was 'a big, big change in her and things have gone very wrong for her'. Alison's mother expressed concern that her speech was becoming slurred, and she had developed a right-sided weakness. She had also fallen over several times but, at the same time, tried to disguise her further deterioration. She had become more sleepy but was determined to maintain her control and independence by refusing to start a course of steroids and have her mother stay with her. In October, Alison fell and fractured her fibula. She was admitted as an in-patient for convalescence and care. She recovered from her fall but continued to deteriorate despite further chemotherapy and treatment.

Terminal period

By December, Alison's deterioration progressed rapidly. She had a poor short-term memory and was no longer able to communicate clearly. Her mobility was limited and she remained unsteady on her feet. Alison agreed to let her mother do more for her and was not averse to her mother staying at her home. She was also finding it painful to remain in the patients' support group and withdrew from it. Much of her anger found an outlet during her music therapy sessions, which were reported as 'very powerful and verging on violence'.

Alison's grief and her resolve to maintain her integrity, despite her losses, appeared to have a sobering and profound impact on the staff. Her nurse said that at times it was difficult for her to absorb the impact of Alison's emotions: 'It is because she also throws everything at me because I am in that role of a nurse and I find it very hard. I come out of a session with Alison sometimes feeling totally shattered and want to cry my eyes out. But she always makes up for it. She always says sorry afterwards. She knows what she has done, that she has really hurt me. She knows that she can use me, but she does, and it takes a bit out of you, but she always afterwards, always, without any doubt, grabs my hand and says "sorry" or just gives me a squeeze, and I know that she is sorry… it helps tremendously.'

Alison's condition deteriorated slowly. In the following months she was admitted, discharged, and readmitted as appropriate. During this time she showed signs of deterioration, such as further loss of coordination, speech and short-term memory. None the less, she was able to spend two weeks with her mother at home before being readmitted. This time, Alison appeared very ill. She died, in the first week of August, without struggle in the presence of her mother and the nurses whom she regarded as her friends. She spent the day before with her friends and family, looking through her photograph album at the things she did earlier in life, amid great laughter and joy.

Case summary 7: Margaret

Age: *70*

Period of contact: *18 months*

Number of conversations with Margaret: *9*

Number of conversations with her nurses: *8*

Living

Admission, medical and social history

Margaret was 70 years old. She was described by her nurse to be prone to mood swings, from being very low to being 'high as a kite'. She was born locally and was an only child. Her father, a cabinet maker, died when she was 14 and she found the experience traumatic. Her mother ran a bed-and-breakfast business and remarried. Margaret described her relationship with her step-father as close. Her relationship with her mother was more distant and they did not get on. Margaret married three times but each marriage ended in divorce. She had developed a 13-year relationship with Trevor, whom she adored. According to Margaret, Trevor had looked after her 'all those years'. Margaret had four children from her first marriage. Sally, her daughter, lived locally and was especially close to her. She described their relationship as being more like sisters. Margaret was brought up a Roman Catholic and confirmed as one. However, she disclosed that 'when I married at 19, I went over to the Church of England'. Margaret believed that she had been helped by God during her life, 'without being really religious'.

Margaret was diagnosed as having breast cancer. This was treated by conservative surgical treatment followed by radiotherapy. Margaret recovered from this and her disease remained stable for seven years until January, when further lymphatic involvement was discovered. She was referred for a series of chemotherapy sessions which eventually led to her referral for palliative care in June. By this time, Margaret was physically unwell, dehydrated and weak, experiencing nausea and vomiting. She was admitted to the in-patient ward in a state of anxiety. Her family thought that she would not survive because of her poor physical state. Her anxiety was made worse by a spell of bad dreams in which she dreamt that pigs and horses were chasing her. After six weeks of treatment and care, Margaret recovered and saw the experience as a 'miracle'. She said that her doctor had saved her life. Her follow-up care included attending the day centre twice a week.

Interim events

In October the same year, Margaret said she felt physically well. She went regularly for her check-ups and would often return to the day centre announcing that she had been cured. She was delighted with her progress and enjoyed her time in the day centre. Margaret would contribute to the social conversations within a group of women. According to her nurses, much of her interaction with them centred on the physical aspects of her care. She presented as someone who was happy to talk superficially about daily issues but would rather not dwell on what she described as 'morbid' matters. She preferred not to talk about the possibility of death or dying and, throughout my conversations with her, Margaret said that she was adopting a positive approach to her life and was convinced that she came through her previous setback through sheer will power and her faith in God.

During the next 12 months, Margaret remained physically stable. Her quality of life was good, and she continued with her social life, enjoying her holidays with Trevor, going out for coffee or a drink with her daughter and friends in the pub. Her self-esteem and confidence in being 'cured' increased. Throughout this time, nursing reports about her progress remained uneventful. Margaret would respond that she was 'fine' and continued to be content. Her inability to accommodate issues that might pose a threat to her remained a key concern for her nurse. The staff felt that underneath her cheerful front she was vulnerable. As her nurse said: 'I do feel a little bit worried if she were to have her cancer come back again, because I think she would be absolutely devastated. She has put all her trust now in being well again. I asked her today if she was thinking of going on holiday, and she said she had such a terrible shock last time she went on holiday that she's very frightened to actually go again.'

On several occasions, when patients with whom she had developed a relationship died, Margaret was very affected. She talked about this to me and decided that in the future she was not going to become close to people. When asked if those deaths reminded her that own life may also be very vulnerable Margaret answered: 'No, no, no... I just carry on. You've got to sort of look forward, haven't you? You haven't got to think back, because I love coming here so much and I know it does us all good, and I had an examination the other day, it was quite by chance with the lady doctor and she said that everything is fine. She can't get over how well I am, and she said that Doctor Murray always says to her that I am a miracle.'

To date, Margaret continues to enjoy a good quality of life and the support and company of the day centre, where her attendance has been reduced to once a week.

Case summary 8: Sheila

Age: *70*

Period of contact: *17 months*

Number of conversations with Sheila: *6*

Number of conversations with her nurses: *6*

Living

Admission, medical and social history

Sheila was a pale 70-year old woman who lived on her own. She was described by her nurse as someone who related in a matter-of-fact way. Sheila was born in the Midlands and was an only child. Most of her childhood was spent at an exclusive boarding school. She enjoyed her time there but would look forward to going back home during the holidays. Her father, whom she adored, died shortly after his retirement from a heart attack, leaving her mother, who died a few years later from cancer. According to Sheila, her mother died a terrible death and suffered for years.

Sheila worked abroad for many years as a welfare officer and retired at 65, returning to live in England. She was married and apparently had a family, but was divorced from her husband. She lived alone and, according to her, she had no friends. Sheila said: 'I've always been very much a lone figure, especially where women are concerned... because I can't tolerate what I call women's talk. I mean, it's too... there's no way I want to go and have coffee and sort of argue about the cost of things in the shops; how many nappies you can get for this, that and the other... I'm just bored. I've no time for fools, no time at all.' Sheila described herself as definitely having a faith, although 'it's been shaken a good many times'. Her idea of Christianity was 'doing' rather than 'going to church and pray'.

In July, Sheila was diagnosed as having inoperable lung cancer with spinal metastases. She had previously had other operations, which included two laminectomies and two laparotomies for bowel obstruction. Fifteen months later, in October, she was referred to the hospice for palliative care and social support following a critical incident when she attempted to commit suicide by taking an overdose of tablets. Sheila felt that she had had enough of 'suffering in constant pain', and had 'lost all her self-esteem, responsibility and independence'. She told her doctor at her first appointment at the hospice that she would attend the day centre on the condition that 'no one were to speak to her about her family'. This message was passed to the staff and, according to them, appeared to be a significant indicator of the way Sheila asserted her control over the health professionals in the months that followed.

Interim events

When Sheila first attended the day centre she was mobile with the help of a stick and said that she was in constant pain. According to her, this was getting her down and led to her 'wanting to end it all'. She was particularly concerned that her body had been changed considerably. Her 'tummy' had become 'bloated', and she was experiencing weakness in her legs, constipation and intractable low back pain.

She spoke openly about her feelings of death and dying in a matter of fact way to me. She was not shocked at being told she had incurable cancer, and with regard to death and dying she said: 'Quite honestly, it is something I have always wanted.' Her reasons for this were apparently 'established sort of 14 years ago, and they have never changed and they never will'. Previous surgery to her lungs and the subsequent bad news that her cancer was inoperable had affected her to the extent that Sheila felt if she had known the outcome she would not have consented to the operation. She saw the time ahead as problematic and had no patience with her own emotions or treatment. 'I have no wish to live. If I die tomorrow it doesn't affect me at all. In fact, I would be very pleased for someone to tell me.'

Throughout the months that followed, Sheila's need to control her situation became more apparent. Her back pain became progressively worse and she was admitted to the in-patient ward for assessment and treatment in March the following year. She was observed to be unwell and was physically weak. This was further exacerbated by episodes of nausea and vomiting. Sheila used a wheelchair to get herself to the smoking room and there she would air her feelings, frustrations, irritability and anger about her treatment and care to other smokers. All the time her anger appeared to be directed at the staff and her treatment and, according to her nurse, on no occasion was it reflected in terms of how she might be really feeling. Attempts to broach this by her nurses were often met with rebuffs and a barrage of complaints about how inept and incompetent the staff had been.

Her nurse and others said that they were frequently at the receiving end of Sheila's moods. She was reported to be rude about the nurses directly or indirectly and played one member of staff off against the other. The nurses responded by trying to lessen her 'rigidity' by providing various activities and also arranging a routine that was predictable and regular for her. However, it became rapidly apparent to the staff that even when mutual agreements had been arrived at, in terms of her care, Sheila would often 'out-manoeuvre' the plans by changing her mind at the last minute. In the months that followed, case conferences were arranged between Sheila and the various teams involved in her care as part of providing consistency and making it clear to everyone the agreed plans.

This 'game' became an established pattern, creating a feeling of failure on the part of her nurses. As one of them said: 'Everybody's complex but, somehow, Sheila is more mysterious. I have a suspicion now, although I might be wrong, that she quite enjoys the dynamics of pushing help away while at the same time being forced to accept it. It becomes almost like a game at times.'

After almost six weeks as an in-patient Sheila slowly recovered and regained her mobility. When I met her there was a difference in how she perceived death and dying. Sheila confessed that since becoming an in-patient she had become 'scared to death of the process of dying'. She went on: 'This is one thing that has changed since I talked to you — I've always accepted death and welcomed it — being so lonely and nobody needing me.' Being in contact with company and forming bonds with other patients and finding that they had died was upsetting for Sheila. During her time as an in-patient Sheila began to care for the others. She continued: 'It felt like losing a relation. There's no way I could be dispassionate about it — I cared too much for them as people. I know I've got terminal cancer. It didn't worry me before. I'm scared that I'll die screaming and shouting. I wonder what's ahead of me. I don't seem to be able to take it.'

This experience was a significant one. Sheila continued to attend the day centre and found it difficult to cope when patients died. She had made a will requesting that she should be buried rather than cremated after her death. When a patient whom she knew died Sheila felt very depressed, saying that it should have been her, because the people who died had families whereas she was on her own. In the following months, her condition plateaued and, although her pain remained constant and chronic, she bore it with fortitude, despite ongoing treatments and epidurals.

Sheila attempted another overdose over Christmas but was unable to go through with it. Three months later she arranged to attend a day centre for people with chronic but not terminal illness and voluntarily reduced her attendance at the hospice from two days to one day a week. When I saw her last she appeared cheerful and looked well. Her nurses subsequently told me that it was part of her plan to 'put off' a mutually agreed arrangement to come in for respite as an in-patient. Apparently, this had been a regular pattern — being extremely nice, only to be followed up by telling staff that she had changed her mind. The following week Sheila cancelled her booked respite admission. To date, her disease appears to have stabilised, and she continues to attend the day centre once a week.

Case summary 9: Ted

Age: *67*

Period of contact: *4 months*

Number of conversations with Ted: *5*

Number of conversations with his nurses: *7*

Place of death: *Acute hospital ward*

Admission, medical and social history

Ted was 67. He had advanced carcinoma of the rectum. His nurses described him as 'a quiet, gentle and reserved man'. Ted was born and brought up locally with his eight brothers. Although raised as 'Church of England', according to Ted religion was not very important to him. He started work as a spinner in a local mill but became a gardener in later years.

Ted married late in life. He was 40 when he met his wife, Emily, in a pub, and married after a long courtship. Emily was 13 years older than Ted and because of their late marriage they had no children. They were a devoted couple and lived in a small bungalow in the country. Ted was initially referred by his GP for additional support in view of his disease progression. His cancer had spread to his liver and a year earlier a partial hepatectomy had been performed. Ted had also required a defunctioning colostomy and radiotherapy to arrest local recurrence of his carcinoma. His disease had spread to the rectal and pelvic areas and Ted experienced perineal pain and bleeding rectally, which had been alleviated by the use of opioids and steroids.

Ted took up the offer of attending the day centre where he could be regularly reviewed for pain relief and symptom control, as well as having some company. Ted's nurses described him as a reticent man who did not create an impression, unlike some other patients. Ted would arrive, 'sit and be', and could easily be forgotten by those around him. He was not naturally chatty nor forthcoming in talking about how he felt. Conversations from him were observed by the nurses as usually minimal, focusing on physical aspects of his illness. When I first approached Ted I found him to be a pleasant and gentle person. He said he was happy for me to chat with him and would not mind participating 'as is' and confided that he was probably not someone who could talk deeply about issues. A nursing entry reported Ted as 'someone who appears stoical about his condition and feels he has had good explanations throughout his illness and is said to be fully in the picture'.

Interim events

A month after my initial contact with Ted he was admitted to the ward for symptom control. His rectal bleeding had worsened, although he was not reporting episodes of rectal pain. He presented with vague symptoms of dizziness, which were diagnosed as 'possibly related to postural hypotension or secondary adrenocortical dysfunction'. During this admission Ted appeared low in mood. On one of my visits he told me that he felt 'down and up'. This caused some concern with the staff. For instance, it was difficult for the nurses and doctors to ascertain whether Ted's 'vagueness' and low mood were a consequence of his illness and required treatment or whether they were more a feature of Ted's personality. As one of the nurses put it: 'Because Ted, in a sense, is so discreet as a person, where the relationship is... there isn't a brick wall between Ted and other people, but a sort of a piece of tissue paper between him and others...' This lack of openness about how he really felt created a barrier, particularly in terms of the nurses' ability to help him effectively face his dying.

At this time, talks with Ted's brother, Tom, revealed that both their parents and three of the other brothers had died of cancer. Tom was awaiting a spinal operation and Ted's other brother, Jack, was nursing his wife, who was dying of cancer. Psychiatric opinion was sought by the doctor who, like the nurses, found it difficult to make a confident diagnosis, although on balance they felt that an antidepressant should be prescribed. Ted agreed, although in the long term the real effects of the antidepressant appeared minimal. Ted also experienced dizzy spells, nausea and vomiting and was often tired. Short home trips were organised for him and Emily continued to visit. Both Ted and Emily wanted him very much to be at home. Eventually this was arranged and Ted was discharged home with back-up support in January, to be followed up by a Macmillan nurse. Ted chose to remain at home and never used the day centre facilities again, even though the offer remained open to him.

I visited Ted in mid-February at his home with the Macmillan nurse. Ted and Emily appeared happy together and were a loving couple, with an endearing sense of humour, teasing each other gently in our company. Ted appeared cheerful, although he had lost more weight and was pale and breathless on walking. Emily showed us round her bungalow and was full of pride. She also mentioned to us that, although Ted enjoyed the day centre, he felt that it was a bit too much of an effort to make the trip at the moment.

Terminal period

In early April Ted was referred to the acute hospital as an emergency by his GP. He was uraemic and consequently admitted to an acute surgical ward. According to the nurse who looked after him on admission, Ted was physically unwell. He was incontinent of urine and had a copious offensive rectal discharge, but was conscious and able to communicate. He was in considerable pain, which distressed the nurses on the ward. As his nurse put it: 'What I found most upsetting was when we were turning him, because he just froze and I thought he was going to start screaming out.' Feelings of guilt about the lack of knowledge and ability to alleviate Ted's pain were expressed by the nurses.

Eventually, the doctors in the acute ward discussed with the palliative care team a regime of pain relief. Five days after admission Ted's pains were largely alleviated through intravenous infusion of diamorphine. I found him barely conscious. My notes read: 'I entered the ward, and asked to see where Ted was and was told that he was in room 9. This happened to be at the top of the ward, a side-room on its own, the first room as one walks into the ward. There Ted lay. He looked absolutely white, he smelt, a pillow was on the floor, the sheets were rumpled and he was wet, incontinent. The scene was one of clinical sterility. He looked pale, unshaven and his mouth was open. His eyes were closed and he was connected to diamorphine and cyclizine pumps. I went up and touched him and reminded him that it was me, Gina, visiting him, and he responded. His eyes twitched and he looked at me, and I felt he did recognise me.'

Together with the nurse looking after Ted, I returned to his room, and this time we asked whether he was in pain or discomfort, to which he responded, barely audibly, that he was not. We washed Ted and made him comfortable and I sat and listened to the nurse, who was distressed. Ted was dying from a necrotic tumour that had begun to penetrate from his rectum. He died the following day, alone, in a side-ward, much to the distress of the nurse looking after him, who wanted to be present but happened to be out of the room. The nurses' impression of Ted's last few moments were that he remained strong-willed, very alert and fighting until the very end.

Case summary 10: Alan

Age: *82*

Period of contact: *8 months*

Number of conversations with Alan: *6*

Number of conversations with his nurses: *5*

Place of death: *Hospice*

Referral, medical and social history

Alan was 82 years old. He had been married to Dorothy for 56 years. They had two children and two grandchildren. Alan was born and brought up locally and was one of four boys in the family. As a young boy he had attended church regularly and his faith was important to him. He went to the local school and as a young man worked in a car factory, making seats, until he retired.

Alan was tall and looked much younger than his age. According to him, apart from a couple of traumatic accidents (one of which resulted in an amputation of his right leg and use of a permanent leg prosthesis) he had always enjoyed relatively good health. Therefore, when he was diagnosed with carcinoma of the rectum it was a big shock to him and his wife. The tumour was inoperable and he was given a permanent colostomy.

Alan was referred in June for palliative care as his disease progressed. He was experiencing rectal pain, bleeding and discharge. His GP wrote that Alan was 'probably entering another phase of his illness where he may well benefit from additional support from the hospice team'. Alan therefore came for a visit to the day centre and was happy to take up the offer of attending regularly.

He enjoyed the activities of the day centre, participating in games of dominoes and exchanges of stamps. He was an avid stamp collector. Known as 'Gentleman Alan' by the nurses, he appeared shy and private, particularly when exposing his body during nursing interventions. Alan would request that a man attend to him in such matters and confessed that he found using pads to cope with the rectal discharge rather humiliating. Although Alan presented as a shy person, he also had a flirtatious side to him. His nurse reported that this was directed in a playful manner to a couple of the nurses who looked after him and provided an insight into another aspect of his personality not immediately obvious. Alan was able to hold conversations, but usually about specific matters. He appeared to choose the people he spoke to carefully and did not want to be of any trouble to anyone. Alan was seen by the nurses as someone who was aware of his cancer and, although initially shocked, he was able to live with it as he felt it was inevitable, particularly in view of his age.

Interim events

The months following his referral saw little change until the next year in May. Alan's attitude towards his illness was very matter of fact — in his words, he might live for another two to three or 10-15 years. In May, Alan's wife died suddenly, following an unexpected stroke, under sad circumstances. Alan and Dorothy had been married for 56 years and were devoted to each other. However, the night before Dorothy died they had had a row and did not make up. Consequently, Alan experienced feelings of guilt and sorrow and was distressed, blaming himself for his wife's death. This event appeared significant. Alan's nurses observed that he began to lose the will to live and never revealed the playful side of himself again. He lost his sparkle for life, was often tearful and seemed a lonely and sad figure. Alan found himself having to cope not only with the grief of facing his own mortality but also with the loss of his wife and their life together. He said: 'I wish I were dead' and began to express thoughts of suicide. He missed his wife profoundly.

The response of the nurses was to provide consistent and realistic support. In the weeks and months that followed, Alan coped for the first time with cooking, ironing and washing and living on his own. He said that he and his wife had always felt that he would be the one to die first and his wife's death was therefore a terrible shock. Alan's despair was profound and in the subsequent months, although he was able to cope well with daily living activities, his grief for his wife was inconsolable. The offer of formal bereavement support was declined, although Alan was happy with the idea of a befriending volunteer who would visit him at home. His primary nurse from the day centre also kept a close watch on him and visited him as appropriate.

Alan was admitted to the ward twice during this time for symptom control. His disease progressed slowly, with signs of deterioration, albeit gradual — such as being incontinent of urine at night. Alan expressed his worries of being a burden to his children when he could no longer look after himself. His concerns centred around not knowing for certain what arrangements had been made and at the same time not wanting to be perceived as a 'scrounger'. Alan said he could not afford to go into a nursing home.

The weeks before Christmas were reported by the staff to be an especially sad time for Alan. Respite admission was booked for him in November, this particular desire being picked up by a member of the day centre team. This wish was put across subtly by Alan who said that he did not want to be a burden to his children.

I visited him just before Christmas and noticed a substantial change. He was pale and had lost weight. His room in the ward was neat and tidy and he told me he made his own bed and was pleased he had a side-room, as there was privacy when he needed to change his colostomy. He was glad to be on the ward, rather than in one of his children's homes, because he did not need to worry about how to dispose his colostomy bags. He was thoughtful and close to tears when we talked about Christmas. He said that the only thing he would have liked for Christmas was to have his wife back.

Terminal period

Christmas day was an emotional time for Alan. His nurse reported that he spent a long time chatting with her and remarked that this was the first Christmas he had spent without his wife. He wanted to be with Dorothy and expressed openly that he wanted to die. Physically, there were no indications that Alan's death was imminent. However, he deteriorated rapidly after Christmas. He contracted a urinary tract infection and the accompanying symptoms of feeling cold, shivery, weak and dizzy. He became breathless and died, without struggle, five days later, in the presence of his son and daughter. His death and rapid deterioration came as surprise to me and the nurses who saw Alan at or just before Christmas.

Case summary 11: James

Age: *67*

Period of contact: *2 months*

Number of conversations with James: *4*

Number of conversations with his nurses: *4*

Place of death: *Hospice*

Admission, medical and social history

James was a 67-year-old retired bank personnel manager and easily engaged people in conversation. He was born in the south of England and grew up with his brother Richard. James later pursued a career in banking and married Joan. A few years after marriage, their first son John was born, followed by Mark. John and Mark both subsequently married and lived quite a distance from their parents. The family were described by the staff as close and kept in touch with each other. James was brought up a Methodist but attended Church of England services regularly with his wife. He had always enjoyed music, the arts, walking and swimming.

Shortly after James's retirement, he was diagnosed as having Parkinson's disease. This was followed by a diagnosis of cancer of the prostate, for which James received surgery, followed by hormonal therapy. This news was upsetting for James and his wife, who felt that much of their hopes for their retirement years had been dashed. In September, James's cancer had spread to his bones and there was evidence of spinal cord compression. James presented with pain, loss of mobility and increasing nocturia. He was also muddled at times, had put on weight and had to use a wheelchair and Zimmer frame to get around. He was referred to the hospice for support and palliative care.

In mid-January the following year, James took up the offer of coming to the day centre as part of social support and ongoing medical and nursing care. The impressions of the nurses may be summed up by the following: 'He was a man who, for want of a better word, was a gentleman, a polite man, a caring man. Somebody with a great sense of fun. Somebody who at one point, I think, worked in the City. From what I gather, what might appear to be the stuffiness of working in the City ran parallel to doing other things such as swimming in the Serpentine. I was told about when he once did that and came back to find his trousers had been stolen and travelled back on the train wearing his shirt, tie, jacket and swimming trunks.'

Interim events

On his first visit to the day centre, James disclosed to his nurse his thoughts of his goals during this period of his care. He wanted very much to walk again and was keen to have physiotherapy and do some swimming. However, his two main goals were to be alive to see the birth of his two grandchildren. The first of these, according to James, had been achieved. He was told in October that he had only six weeks to live but had survived past that time to see his first grandchild born in December. His next hope was to be alive to see his second grandchild, whose birth was expected in May the following year.

During the next three visits to the day centre James appeared to be making progress physically. He enjoyed his swimming and with support was beginning on a mobilising programme. His pain was also alleviated. I talked to him during this time and he was keen to participate in my study. He expressed his sadness about his imminent death and wished that he had more time to be able to do some of the things he had planned for his retirement. He was concerned about his wife and family and wondered whether he was letting them down.

In mid-March, James appeared weaker and experienced some nausea and vomiting. He had also developed a chest infection and was treated with antibiotics by his GP. He missed a few visits to the day centre but resumed his routine at the beginning of April. He looked and felt much better and was more mobile. However, the following week James deteriorated and was admitted as an in-patient to the ward. He was to remain there until his death three weeks later.

Terminal period

On arrival, the staff reported that both James and Joan were distressed. Joan had not slept for the past few days and James was tearful and distressed about his dying. His nurse spent time with him and, during the next couple of hours, James was reported as calmer, less muddled and able to go to sleep.

He spent a restless night, in part disturbed by having to have his bed linen changed as a result of his incontinence. He was also anguished, asking the night nurse 'if he was dying and was he going mad?' James continued to be in this state from time to time the following morning and appeared to experience flashbacks to his childhood, calling for his mother and brother Richard. He was calmer when Joan was with him.

Throughout this admission, James continued to deteriorate at a steady pace. His mood and lucidity continued to fluctuate. His speech was muddled and on occasions it was clear that he was struggling with his confusion. Much of the nursing care and treatment were undertaken in partnership with Joan, who would often stay overnight at the hospice. Joan remained the key person and link between James and the nurses. James was tearful on occasions and 'terrified of dying', and this was seen as linked to a number of issues. James said that he would 'like to be alive in two years' time'. Statements such as 'I'm dying and I really want to be up and dancing with my grandchildren' were expressed between tears. His grief at the multiple losses he was experiencing was very vivid. James's anguish was also linked with religious questions of whether his life had been 'good enough' and whether there was an after-life. Moreover, it also appeared that, beneath the surface, issues related to James's childhood and his past relationship with his brother were causing him some guilt and distress.

When these feelings were expressed, James's nurses, working together with Joan, were able to help James settle some of his disquiet about those issues. His priest came and anointed James with oil, which seemed to bring some calm. His brother Richard was contacted and James was able to spend time alone with him. His children and grandchild visited and were able to talk to him. According to his nurse, he had also expressed a desire to be cremated and for his wife to scatter his ashes over a particular mountain where they had walked together.

James continued to deteriorate and would dwell on certain aspects of things that bothered him. On one such occasion, the nurse who was with him and his wife remarked on the lovely relationship his wife had with him. Joan was able to tell James: 'You've sorted things out with Richard, you've sorted things out in the past, all you need to do now is to exist for the pleasure of your family.'

On the 12th day of his admission, while Joan was out, James's condition deteriorated further. He became agitated, crying out in pain. After an hour's deliberation and waiting for Joan to return, it was decided that for James' comfort it was necessary to go ahead with an injection of diamorphine and midazolam. This decision had to be taken without consultation with Joan. The medication was reported by the staff to have good effect; James was calmer and relieved of his pain. However, he could never be roused sufficiently to be able to talk to his wife again. He died two days later, quite rapidly, in her presence. According to his nurse, his eyes were 'half open and he appeared to be in "slight distress" but slowly calmed down, with Joan holding his hand'.

His death was reported by the nurse to have aroused some misgivings with Joan. She expressed feelings of guilt that she had not been not around at the critical moment when she felt that James needed her. Moreover, she confided that there had been some 'unfinished emotional business' between them. It was only in the latter days of their marriage that they had begun to communicate on an emotional level. As a result, Joan expressed regret that she had not done this sooner.

Case summary 12: Peter

Age: *48*

Period of contact: *6 months*

Number of conversations with Peter: *6*

Number of conversations with his nurses: *6*

Place of death: *Hospice*

Referral, admission and social history

Peter was 48 years old. He used to work as a bookbinder. He lived with his second wife Joyce and between them they had three children — Sam and Amanda, from their previous marriages, and Ben, a nine-year-old. Peter was an only child, brought up in 'religious surroundings'. His father had been a church hall caretaker and the family lived for most of their lives in a church house. According to Peter, he was not religious and was ambivalent about God, despite coming from a religious background. His views about this were openly expressed. He had had quite a happy childhood. Peter's relationship with his father became closer and stronger once he left home and he felt that he was closer to his father than his mother. At the time of his admission to hospice care his father had already died and his mother was in a nursing home.

Peter developed multiple sclerosis when he was 25 and had to give up work seven years later. At about this time, his first marriage deteriorated. Because of contracting a chronic illness at an early age, Peter said he had adopted a philosophical approach to life in general. At the age of 46 he was diagnosed with rectosigmoid carcinoma, and two years later he was referred to the day centre for palliative care and social support. Peter's nurses described him as someone with a positive approach to his situation, despite his age and the losses he had experienced. For example, he talked about seeing the end of full-time employment as simply providing an opportunity for a different way of living. Peter and his wife had set up a smallholding rearing 'chickens, ducks and goats and other bits and pieces'. Talking to one of the nurses, Peter explained his outlook on life: 'I see a cup as being half full, not half empty.' According to reports from the staff, Peter presented as someone who was very knowledgeable about his situation.

Interim events

A few weeks after coming to the day centre, Peter was referred to the acute hospital by his doctor for further surgery on his tumour. In June he underwent a course of radiotherapy and chemotherapy to reduce the tumour size in preparation for the forthcoming surgery. The days leading up to the surgery were reported by his nurse to be difficult ones for Peter and Joyce. In their own ways, both of them had felt that the operation was their hope for a normal future. Although the disease had not spread to his peritoneal cavity and liver, the surgery confirmed the presence of a tumour that had clearly not been 'downstaged', despite preoperative radiotherapy.

Peter's nurse reported that this period of time also provided a glimpse into how Peter responded to news that was not good, but not surprising either. The imminence of death appeared to have become more real to Peter. For instance, he wrote a farewell letter to Joyce, and during conversations with the nurses he appeared to test out their responses to his condition. He told one of them that he felt the idea of future surgery, possibly in a year or even five year's time, put to him by the surgeon, was unrealistic. Peter said that the doctor was trying to make him feel better and at that moment he was not ready to die.

At the same time, Peter was observed by the staff as very resourceful in mobilising support and using staff to his advantage in order to lessen additional burdens for his wife. Peter's capacity to mobilise support took place on the first day postoperatively. Doctors and nurses from the hospice (including me) were contacted by the nurse from the acute ward. All the key people knew that Peter's wish was to return to the hospice for convalescence and not to go home. This was subsequently arranged and Peter was admitted to the hospice following his discharge from the acute hospital. Peter appeared very much in control, despite recovering from major surgery.

During his convalescence, Peter maintained a certain amount of hope that 'things could still be done', although he was aware that the news from his operation were not good. He continued with a positive approach in general during his convalescence. His condition plateaued for the next couple of months with gradual deterioration. Throughout this time, Peter attended the day centre regularly. According to the nurse caring for him, he had chosen to be in denial about his situation and during conversations would talk about things that would occur over the next 10 years. This created distress for his wife, as Peter seemed unable to talk about his condition openly with her. Ben, their nine-year-old son, had started to ask Joyce questions about Peter's illness and this added further to Joyce's distress.

In September Peter's physical deterioration became more evident and he was admitted to the ward for respite and symptom control. Peter's stepdaughter Amanda was getting married and the events in the days that followed revolved around her wedding. This created additional stress for Joyce and was an emotional period of time which veered between happiness and sadness for the whole family. This situation continued after the wedding, with Joyce requiring considerable support from the staff. On a daily basis, Peter continued to cope with his condition by talking about things other than what was happening to him. This carried on, with the nurses respecting his wish not to talk about his dying while at the same time supporting his distressed wife.

In October it was reported by nurses that Peter had shown a significant shift in attitude. He suddenly wanted to talk and ask questions about his dying and death. He asked to speak to a particular nurse whom he had grown to trust. Peter wanted to know what would happen when he died and, according to him, until then no one had mentioned cancer to him. However, according to the nurse this was the first time Peter had used the word cancer in her presence. During the next two days Peter talked openly to Joyce about his death and dying and about how to prepare their son for the event. Peter talked to his doctor and nurses and said that he was ready to die. There appeared to be a sense of relief all round for the staff caring for Peter and his family, but also intense and continuous grief for Joyce, who wept with the nurses and found it difficult to stay with Peter to watch him dying slowly.

Terminal period

Three days after he declared that he was ready to die and finding that he was still living, Peter apparently reverted back to previous form. The nurses on the ward reported that he had started to talk about seeing his son growing up and renewing his driving licence. Peter continued to attend the day centre in his emaciated state, which distressed staff and the other patients around him. The picture he presented was of a living death and 'horrendous', according to the day centre nurses. Peter had become very weak and was close to death. He was also jaundiced, pale, sleepy and had a short memory span. His death was imminent. The usefulness of the day-centre facilities to him was raised but Peter was spared further discussion of this. He died quietly the following morning at 8.30am, without struggle, in the presence of nurses. The day before his death, Joyce had taken Peter out into the hospital grounds in a wheelchair. At the time of his death, Joyce and Ben were at home. Peter donated his body to medical science for research and his wish for a memorial service (rather than a funeral service) was met, attended by staff and family.

6. "Taking each day as it comes"

CROSS-CASE COMPARISONS: ANALYSIS OF ACCOUNTS OF PATIENTS' EXPERIENCES AND THOSE OF THEIR NURSES

This chapter presents a cross-case comparison and analysis of the accounts of patients' and their nurses. Extracts of their accounts from interviews and from my field notes (including background data) are used to illuminate the interplays that occurred. The data are presented in the form of three major themes that have emerged as a result of the coding process:

- protecting and controlling;

- watching and waiting;

- holding on and letting go.

The first theme, protecting and controlling, featured continually throughout the patients' dying trajectory. The second, watching and waiting, increasingly occurred as the patients' physical condition deteriorated. The third theme, holding on and letting go, featured in the terminal phase. Metaphors used by the patients (such as 'Taking each day as it comes', 'Past my sell by date', and 'I don't know how to die') have been retained as headings to organise the data relating to each of the themes, as they represent the dominant concepts that appeared important to the patients during the course of the study.

TAKING EACH DAY AS IT COMES

For much of the time covered by this study, each patient was involved in being part of everyday activities. This metaphor 'taking each day as it comes' recalls the constant need for dying patients to carry out the normal activities of daily living. Patients often told me they take each day as it comes, which involved carrying on with housework, such as washing and ironing, mowing the grass and experiencing the excitements of holidays, weddings and births. However, central to the dying person's life is that much of 'taking each day as it comes' is punctuated by a programme of treatments and admissions, feeling well on some days and unwell on others. This is reminiscent of the concept of a treatment calendar reflected in Schou's (1993) work, which described the various treatments faced by cancer patients.

The everyday-life activities of the dying can therefore be seen as dependent on their physical well-being and go beyond accommodating and incorporating normal life events. It has much to do with the other aspects of the dying person's life, such as treatments, admissions and living with a range of losses including, finally, the experience of death.

These rather distinct everyday-life activities of the dying are shared in nurse-patient encounters by a process of face-to-face social exchange of information, contribution and participation.

From the data analysis it emerged that dying patients appeared to employ various strategies to protect themselves, their families and the nurses by exerting control over everyday-life activities and in accommodating treatments that were provided. Protecting and controlling featured as the dominant theme throughout the patients' dying trajectory, particularly relating to the way they exercised personal control and control over others during mundane aspects of everyday life but also through a demanding and emotionally trying sequence of investigations, treatments and care.

Protecting and controlling

An important component of this interplay of strategies is the act of 'protecting'. This has emerged from both the patient and nurse data and can be classified into three main categories: protecting kin, patient and nurse protecting each other, and protecting self. These three categories, while individually distinct can also intertwine. In my observation they occurred at varying times and to varying degrees and were context-related. Protecting occurred in different ways, for different reasons and at different levels. For instance, the function of protecting others was not always based on altruism. It appeared to serve a fundamental and personal need of protecting the individuals themselves.

In this study, 'control' seemed to a be dynamic process and reflected the way in which the patient chose to manage the treatment or care aspects of their dying. Central to this was the control exerted by patients over how remissions, setbacks, progressive losses and dying were perceived and accommodated at critical junctures. This appeared to be expressed through talking and, in so doing, making known to others their individual concerns, fears or wishes (perceived as being 'open about dying'), or not talking and, therefore, not making these concerns known (that is, not being open about dying). When viewed as a spectrum, protecting and controlling are related opposites, occupying different ends of the same dimension.

Protecting kin

This stemmed primarily from caring about loved ones and was expressed by most of the patients through the work of 'worry'. During our conversations, patients often talked about their worries and concerns about burdening family members, either with having to care for them or with personal worries about their condition and their feelings about dying. For instance, when we talked about how he coped with the thought of death and dying, Ian (case 4) replied: 'Well, that is at the back of your mind, but what worries me more is when I say "cope with it", I try not to burden the family more than is necessary because obviously they worry, and this in a way I don't like, because I don't like to think of them worrying about me... Obviously when I was having treatment, they were worried, I was worried... it was a good outcome, which was good, but even then there was still a certain amount of worry. When I see how it affected my family, nobody ever complained. My wife has never complained, even to this day, or the children, but I know signs that have sort of come out that they were worrying within themselves and this is my biggest problem.'

For those who were open about their dying, the act of talking openly was sometimes used indirectly as a means to assert control over admissions and care. This served to protect the family from being burdened by the patient's care but, more importantly, maintained personal self-worth and autonomy. Patients often engaged key carers in talk, conveying their needs and wishes, as in the case of the patient below (case 10), who was worried about where and how he was going to be cared for when he could no longer do that himself. At the time of this conversation, Alan's wife, who had always looked after him, had just died suddenly and Alan was having to fend for himself.

Case 10 (Alan)

GC: Alan, you know the last time we talked — it must have been six weeks ago, something like that — our conversation was really about that you were a bit worried about what was going to happen to you. How are you at the moment? Is that still in your mind?

A: Oh yes, it's bound to be in my mind, because you see, my daughter is a full-time teacher, so obviously she couldn't be with me and if I went there, I couldn't come here, and my daughter-in-law is practically a full time teacher, and she has got two small children and she lives out in the country where I would never be able to come here. The point is, what happens to me when I am incapable of changing this?

GC: 'This' meaning the colostomy bag?

A: Yes. At the present it is quite alright. I don't see any trouble but the stoma nurse has given me an explanation of a new system they have got, the irrigation system, which is, you don't wear a bag, and it lasts from 24 hours to 48 hours and it does what it says, irrigation. It cleans it all out and it takes at least an hour and you have got to be in a house where there is more than one toilet because if you are in the toilet for an hour, obviously somebody would want to use that toilet, and that would be impossible because it is a complicated job. Evidently it pumps something and another one pumps it out straight into the toilet. That is alright if I was somewhere where there is two bathrooms. At the present time, I'm thinking about it.

GC: Can I ask you another question? Where would you like to be when you can no longer cope with things yourself?

A: It's not where I would like to be, it's what would happen because I could never afford to go into a nursing home because I have only got a small amount of money. Not much, which with what I draw now, enables me to look after myself, but if I went into a home, it has got to be somewhere with somebody. Well, I just can't understand what I am going to do and that is a worry.

GC: Have you talked about this to anyone? The nurses?

A: I have spoken to Marianne and Sandra and I have had a chat with Jenny, the stoma nurse, but at the moment I am alright. How long I am going to be, I don't know. From what they told me before, they would look after me here, but I can't see how they would have me here just to do that.

By making his fears and wishes known, as Alan became less well the nurses were able to respond. Admissions were planned and he received in-patient care as required. This became particularly important as Christmas approached. Alan was concerned that his grief for his wife and his illness would affect his children's celebration, so a bed was booked for him over the holiday period, sparing Alan the additional worries of burdening his family.

Similarly, Peter (case 12) who underwent further surgery to his tumour, showed his capacity to mobilise support by making his wishes of convalescing at the hospice (rather than at home) known. This took place on the first postoperative day. Doctors and nurses from the hospice were contacted by the nurse on the acute ward. Peter talked to key people (including me) and said openly that he did not want to be an additional burden to his wife and wanted to be admitted back to the hospice. He achieved this and the following is a conversation two weeks after his admission.

Case 12 (Peter)

GC: Peter, it is now two weeks since your operation. I would really like to know how you are feeling at this moment and what your thoughts are.

P: Well, I think because I have had the first operation I knew what to expect, or thought I did. Things were obviously different with this operation. Nothing ever goes quite the same but I had some idea of how things would happen and how I would feel. Looking back now, it is very difficult to try and explain but I feel stronger in my understanding of myself. Although people say that I've got a very laid-back attitude I still somehow feel that I need to be in control because when you have the operation everybody else controls you, with the drugs and with the bits and pieces, and you really have no personal control over your feelings about anything. Someone says: 'Right, now we'll turn you over,' and they try to turn you over. You can't say: 'I don't want to turn over.' I wouldn't like to say I'm now fitter, but I'm getting back to being in control of my situation, more able to cope, and Joyce would be more able to cope. She has had more help through the hospice, through their general caring attitude than the home assistant gave her when I came out of hospital the first time. I was dumped in bed at home, couldn't really move, but this time things are much better.

Peter's nurse, Brenda, made this observation:

B: I was interested to observe our 'patient' and 'nurse' roles. Communication was very easy and I felt quite equal and I was not aware of any prohibitive boundaries between us. Peter made it very easy to build up a relationship. However, when I stood back and reflected on our time spent together I often felt I had not achieved very much. Perhaps it was because I didn't have very much to offer Peter. I observed this frequently and came to the conclusion that Peter had now had many years of learning how to communicate with professionals and I think he had perfected this technique, so that he would be able to meet his own needs, using us as vehicles. As the time passed by and the whole multidisciplinary team became involved this became more evident. This, I feel, was not a bad thing, but interesting to see how a patient could conduct the professionals to meet his needs like a grand chess master moving the pieces on the board.

In contrast, patients who appeared 'not open about dying' and the act of not talking openly was sometimes a combination of the person's condition and personality. The nurses caring for such a person — for example, Ted (case 9) — found it difficult to know whether they had met his needs. Ted was not very articulate and rarely talked about how he felt. The following extracts provide his nurses' descriptions of him.

Case 9 (Kevin: Ted's nurse)

K: Ted, in a sense, is so discreet a person that the relationship is, in a sense... there isn't a brick wall between Ted and other people but a sort of a piece of tissue paper between him and other people, and it is very hard to record Ted's day or document in the nursing notes without being repetitive. In a strange sort of way while, on the one hand because Ted is a human being, because he is a person, you could write lots and lots and lots, on the other hand, day to day, there isn't a vast amount that can be written.

Case 9 (Jan: Ted's nurse)

GC: With all the things you have highlighted, how does that affect your caring for him? Does it make it challenging or difficult?

J: I think it makes it difficult, and there's a few reasons why. I think physically Ted is independent and we've had other people in our team who have been more physically dependent, and so as a result of that have had more of our time. So I think there is a tendency for Ted to be neglected when it comes to time being spent with him and because of that there's been perhaps a difficulty in establishing a trustful relationship with him. So I think that's posed a problem, and I think also because Ted is a very private person, he doesn't talk openly about his feelings about what's going on, it is quite difficult then to know what's going on because he doesn't openly talk about it and that's his right to be like that, but that does make it difficult, I find.

At other times, the 'act of not talking openly' was described by some patients as not wanting to upset loved ones more than is necessary. This is illustrated by the conversation I conducted with Carol.

Case 2 (Carol)

C: My father died when I was 10. He died of cancer too. He had a brain tumour. So it kind of runs in the family.

GC: Have you managed to speak openly about this to your son?

C: Certain things, but he gets upset, so I try to stay off it.

This aspect of controlling (by not talking openly) as part of protecting occasionally gave rise to tension and distress, particularly when the spouse or children expressed the need to know the wishes of the individual. In my conversations with the nurses, when this occurred the nurse looking after that particular individual appeared caught in the middle. On the one hand, the nurses wanted to respect the wishes of the dying person. On the other hand, watching the impact of that action on the family, as well as having to provide support equally to patient and family members, was reported as emotionally difficult to sustain over a period of time.

Various strategies, such as providing cues and chances for patients to air anger and inner fears, were observed as being used by nurses to create opportunities of breaking this tension. This involved 'testing the water' with the patient and relied to a large extent on the relationship between nurse and patient. Sometimes the assistance of another colleague, who was perceived to know the family better, was sought to act as a go-between for the patient and family. To protect their loved ones from being burdened by worry some patients did not openly express to their spouse or family personal thoughts about dying and matters regarding funeral and financial arrangements. This appeared to lead to tension between the patient and their family members. In Carol's case (case 2) this tension increased as her death became imminent. The account below demonstrates how an in-patient nurse requested the help of Tina, a Macmillan nurse, (who knew Carol and her son well) to act as a go-between in breaking the tension.

Case 2 (Tina: Carol's nurse)

GC: Tina, tell me a little about what happened before Carol's death.

T: On around the Tuesday or Wednesday, one of her primary nurses, Sally, came to me and said that she was very worried that Mike had asked her if she could find out from Carol what Carol's wishes were for her ashes after she died. Sally felt that she couldn't do this and came to me to ask if I could do it. Mike had expressed that he was unable to ask his mother. So on the Wednesday afternoon, I spoke with Mike and we both went to the bedside together and I said to Carol I had come to ask her something on behalf of Mike, as it was very painful for Mike to ask her, and that was to ascertain just what her wishes were about her ashes. Carol's reaction was that she had expressed a desire in the past for them to go to America, but that now she was going to leave the decision up to Mike. We then discussed (the three of us) that Mike's needs may be that he might have the needs of having somewhere to go to put flowers on, or whatever, and Carol agreed with this and it became very painful for Mike. He did a lot of crying and had to leave the bedside. I then went and talked to Mike about it and, after he left the hospice, I went back to Carol's bedside to ask her again without Mike being there if that was really what her wishes were and again she said that she would leave it to Mike.

The need to balance caring for the patient and family was perceived by nurses as a fine art and, on occasions, divided loyalties seem to have occurred. This seemed to be dependent on the experience of the nurse and the extent to which patients concerned were willing or able to disclose private thoughts and feelings. The intensity of grief being expressed was also pertinent. Although most nurses confided that it was easier to care for patients who were open and willing to talk about their dying and needs, not all patients would talk openly about their fears and thoughts about dying. This situation appeared confounded when close family members wanted to talk but the patient felt unable to respond at that time. For instance, unlike his wife Joyce, who expressed her grief openly throughout his dying, Peter (case 12) adopted a calm and deliberately philosophical approach and seldom talked openly to his wife. When this occurred, nurses acting as go-betweens found themselves having to shift the balance of emotional support towards Joyce, who was then perceived by them as needing extra support. The following account illustrates the nature and impact of this emotional support on the nurse caring for Peter and his wife.

Case 12 (Brenda: Peter's nurse)

B: Joyce rang yesterday, very distressed on the phone, more distressed than usual, really saying she couldn't cope. There were long silences on the telephone when she was just crying and I think it had built up over the previous two days and she didn't want him to come here. I was trying to say I understood her problems because she had always been very happy coming here. Joyce did come in later, because what she said to me was that she couldn't face seeing Peter here. I had a message from the front desk to say that she was staying in the car and couldn't come in, would I go and talk to her?

GC: What did she tell you?

B: Well, her father had died here, although when she had previously been in both her Macmillan nurse and I and her had been on to the ward and seen the room where her father had died and it wasn't a completely new area. She knew this was happening, it wasn't out of the blue. I think it was that everything was coming to a head and because it was yet another change. All those things she had been pushing down — it was like another thing she had to cope with and it all came up.

GC: Have you been to see Peter?

B: Yes. He is clear, he feels very relaxed, he is very pleased to be here. I went as soon as he arrived yesterday. I eventually did take Joyce to see him yesterday and I have been this morning. He is calm and understands what is going on. He said to me he felt Joyce was distressed because of the change. He is such a contrast.

GC: Have they been able to talk quite openly with each other?

B: Joyce feels she hasn't been able to talk to Peter, and that is something that I have encouraged her to do. I sat with her in the car for 20 minutes before she eventually did come in and have a cup of tea yesterday afternoon, and then eventually she definitely wanted to see Peter but it took her a long time and she went in and burst into tears and they had time together and then went off again.

At each particular critical juncture of Peter's illness, Joyce turned to the nurses for support. The extract below demonstrates again the impact of Joyce's grief and the response of the same nurse, following more bad news as a result of further surgery conducted on Peter.

Case 12 (Brenda: Peter's nurse)

B: The next day I was visited by Joyce. We sat together and talked about the week's events. It was obvious from observing her that she was in complete overload from having to cope with so much. She was very frightened and tearful and feeling that there was no support for her. She was having to reassess her relationship and role. She expressed frustration and said she would end up being in the same position she had been in when she first met Peter, that is as a struggling one-parent family. I stayed with Joyce and just listened. There was little I could do to take away her grief, but I felt it was important for Joyce to verbalise her fears and frustrations. Being of a similar age to Joyce, and also being a mother, allowed me to be able to imagine myself in her position, and while this is painful and tiring, as there is no apparent end to the situation, it allowed me to feel empathy, and I hope that Joyce felt that support was available to her.

'Protecting kin' therefore occurred between patient and family and nurse and family. Patients appeared to engage in this process through the act of worry and fear of burdening family members. Personal control over this matter was exercised through the work of 'talking openly' or 'not talking openly'. This sometimes created tension between patient and family. Nurses acting as go-betweens often tried to break this tension with patient and family and for another nursing colleague. Emotional support was shifted towards kin in the case of family members who expressed distress and grief often, with a profound impact on the nurse.

Protecting each other

'Protecting kin' was not solely confined to patient and family situations. Patients and nurses also appeared to protect each other. Protecting patients was usually performed by nurses as part of preventing and controlling embarrassment as deterioration occurred. Protecting nurses was expressed in several ways: through praise for the kindness and support shown by them and putting on a brave face in adverse circumstances. In analysing the cases, the latter appeared to be significant in the way nurses and patients related to one another and served to contribute to further understanding of how the expression of feelings could be enabled in a manner that is safe.

Jane (case 3) was an attractive woman with an instant smile, extremely sociable and cooperative towards the nurses. She would talk openly about her dying. Jane was increasingly confined to her bed because of spinal secondaries causing continuous pain, despite medication. According to Jane, 'analgesics take the edge off, but the pain is always there, niggling.' As I got to know her, I realised that Jane had tremendous inner strength and a great sense of humour. I gathered fairly early on that some of the nurses found Jane difficult to care for because of her smiles and appearance of being brave. For instance, comments from nurses would include: 'Poor Jane. She puts on a brave face but, underneath those smiles, who knows what her real feelings are.'

The incidents below provide two accounts of how Jane put on a brave face to protect staff.

Case 3 (Jane)

Jane was admitted to the ward as part of her respite programme. During this admission her pain was not well alleviated. During the medical round, the consultant and nurse discussed with Jane plans for medication to alleviate her pain. I was present and was aware of the way Jane appeared to smile in spite of the pain she was experiencing in her back. After the consultant had spoken there was a short period of silent reflection. Jane broke this silence, by saying 'don't look so worried, doctor, I'm alright.' She wriggled and winced in pain but gave everyone a beaming smile.

The mismatch between the public and private fronts of how some patients conduct themselves appeared to cause considerable concern for some nurses, particularly when progressive deterioration was apparent. This perception of mismatch was arrived at through the work of watching patients' physical deterioration and the patients' perception and responses to this deterioration. The concern was often privately expressed between nurses, and between nurses and doctors. Some nurses tried to regain an equilibrium of control by breaking this tension; others appeared to let matters take their own course, with the patient remaining in control until a point was reached when the patient's public and private feelings synchronised, such as when it became apparent to them that death was imminent. For instance, during Jane's admission to the in-patient unit, the perceived mismatch between her public and private fronts towards her deterioration caused concern and disquiet among the nurses, as Jane continued to smile and put up a brave front. I interviewed Heather, one of the nurses who had been looking after Jane.

Case 3 (Heather: Jane's nurse)

GC: Heather, what are your worries about Jane?

H: Well, when I was talking to Jane last night she asked me what the tightness in her feet could be, and there was no reason for it, her socks weren't too tight or anything like that, and I asked her what did she think it could be. She said she worries about her legs and I asked whether or not it was part of her back problem. She was distressed about this but was still smiling but yet was crying and I said to her: 'Look Jane, is this one of the things you are concerned about? Is this one of the things you worry about?' Jane said: 'No, nothing much worried me,' and was smiling. And I said: 'I don't believe you, Jane. I think a lot of things worry you but you don't like to worry us with your worries.'

      And I explained that it was her right that she didn't need to tell us if she didn't want to, but I also wanted her to know that we know she is worrying and that we care that she is worrying. She looked at me and seemed to accept that and then changed the subject.

GC: And how did that leave you?

H: That was alright. It was okay because I knew that what I'd said made sense to her and I felt good that I was able to express to her that I knew things were worrying her even though she didn't want to tell us and that she wanted to put on a brave face. I also felt it was good that she also knew that we weren't wanting to drag those worries out if she didn't want to express them. But perhaps now she knew that she could if she wanted to.

For those nurses who felt that the mismatch between public and private fronts was best left to take its own course, relief was expressed when the patient eventually decided to be open about the situation, thus breaking the tension. Despite progressive deterioration, Peter controlled his situation by choosing not to talk openly about his condition, either to his wife or to the in-patient nurses until he felt ready.

Case 12 (Elsa: Peter's nurse)

GC: I hear that Peter is now talking about his dying?

E: Yes, now he's allowed himself to talk. He can be more open than most other patients are because he has missed out all the other stages. He has just got to the stage where he can say what he feels rather than having to protect people. He can be really honest.

GC: Has Peter actually talked to you about his dying?

E: He has never talked to any of the nursing, medical staff or to Joyce about his dying until now. He's used us very much as carers and nothing else, and it's been very much a denial. At the weekend, he was quite poorly and producing melaena, and he could have died, but because he hadn't let go and said what he needed to say he's gotten better and physically he has improved. Now he's waiting for something his body is not ready to do.

GC: How do you, as a nurse caring for him, help him? How do you cope with it?

E: All you can do is listen and be there and give him the support he needs. And if he wants you there, stay, and if he doesn't accept that's his choice, and he might not want to talk with me. He might just want me to do things, carry out physical care and that's it, and that's fine.

Nurses too, made attempts to protect patients as part of preventing and overcoming embarrassment, particularly as progressive losses occurred. Protecting patients in this way is not new and has been previously reported in Lawler's (1991) work on somological nursing. Lawler (p166) observed that nurses used 'minifisms' defined as 'verbal and/or behavioural techniques which assist in the management of potentially problematic situations by minimising the size, significance, or severity of an event'. Similarly, in this study, skilful but subtle means were used to protect patients. This was carried out in a number of situations and in different ways. They included understating situations that were potentially embarrassing (such as when patients were incontinent), and purposefully conducting conversations that did not require long explanations of events or recall when patients were seen to experience poor short-term memory or slurred speech. This style of protecting patients by preventing embarrassment was observed to be subtly disclosed to other staff, so that they too would adopt the same approach.

The act of 'pacing' was another strategy sometimes used by nurses to protect patients from embarrassment. This involved using actions that were set according to the pace of the patient. Pacing, as a process, involves choice of timing and duration of time for the particular action, and these two elements were normally initiated by the nurse.

Alison (case 6) had recently fallen and broken her tibia. She continued to deteriorate slowly and found it particularly difficult watching the changes that were occurring to her body. She was unable to walk and had to use a wheelchair. Alison used the day centre regularly and was well known to the patients and staff. The following is an account of how Alison's nurse helped her to overcome some of her embarrassment in transporting herself in a wheelchair to the day centre.

Case 6 (Debbie: Alison's nurse)

D: She [Alison] actually saw the fact that having a broken leg and having to use a wheelchair as being looked on as a cripple. And that has been something that has really worried Alison all along through her illness — that having seen other people get 'bigger', and that is the steroids, and this is where our [referring to Alison] fear and hate of steroids are. Having now lost the use of her limbs and being in a wheelchair to her is being crippled, and this was a tremendous hurdle she had to get over. Just even getting out of her room... she didn't want to come out of the room in the wheelchair. We slowly tackled this, like I walked her round the outside of the day centre sitting room in the wheelchair first of all and actually just came to the door and we looked at the door and we didn't go any further. We went back and the next time we did come through and when we came through she did then come into the day centre, but couldn't stay too long. She found it very difficult, because everyone was so nice to her, maybe overpoweringly nice, but she did say afterwards: 'They were pleased to see me.' It was nice, but she said: 'I saw them looking at the wheelchair.'

Following this, very gradually Alison overcame some of her embarrassment and was soon transporting herself to the day centre.

These acts of protecting were performed subtly in the course of the patients' and nurses' everyday activities. Although much of this interplay of protecting and controlling was subsumed under the apparent motivation of concern for another, some of these activities indirectly acted as a means of self-protection.

Protecting self

For both patients and nurses the acts of protecting and controlling others can be suggested to be linked to a more private, subconscious intention — that of protecting the self and, in so doing, preventing one's own inner being from disintegrating. Protecting self may be conducted by reconstructing situations (and in so doing redefining self), during and after nurse-patient encounters. A knowledge of the inner self has sometimes been argued as instrumental in providing a basis from which individuals obtain a sense of their being as individuals (Cassell 1991). The instinctive drive and the human make-up to readjust threats to the inner being through a process of reconstructing situations in order to make them less threatening has also been viewed as crucial for individuals' survival.

For the patients, central to protecting self is the assertion of control, through talking or not talking openly about deterioration or dying. As discussed in chapter 1, it was not uncommon for patients who were dying to use denial-like mechanisms as part of coping in order to maintain control, preserve self-esteem and prevent disintegration (Weisman 1972; Rainey 1988). A number of strategies appeared to be used by people to protect the self. Some patients used talk to off-load concerns and worries, others did not talk openly and thus prevented themselves being reminded of their losses. Both actions appeared to affect their nurses in different ways by evoking different responses. Even for those patients who used open talking to protect self, the impact of this on the nurse was dependent on whether the public and private fronts of what was being said and acted were congruent. This is exemplified by cases 1 and 3.

On discovering that her disease was incurable, Susan (case 1) requested to come into the hospice for support in the form of massage, relaxation and having someone to talk to. Throughout her illness, Susan talked openly to the nurses but less so to her family. She often cried and appeared anxious and frightened. Despite the situation being emotionally difficult, Susan's nurses expressed less conflict in Susan's case, as her grief, sadness and anxiety were perceived as appropriate. Her public and private fronts appeared to match.

In contrast, although Jane (case 3) also talked openly about her dying, her public expressions of non-worry and telling others not to worry, as well as projecting a cheerful front, appeared to create more conflicts and tensions with the nurses. This may, however, have enabled Jane to protect her inner, private self. On rare occasions this private self was revealed, but only fleetingly, as in the incident described below.

Case 3 (Jane)

One morning I was working with Sandra. We were both helping Jane to pack her clothes before being discharged. We were chatting to Jane and commented on her sense of humour and cheerfulness. Jane replied: 'You've got to laugh, haven't you? Laugh and the world laughs with you, cry and you cry alone.' Sandra then gently probed Jane by saying: 'Do you find yourself in situations when you cry alone?' Jane answered quietly and sadly: 'Yes, usually at night, by myself' and then, instantly, her face brightened up with the most attractive smile.

The two cases serve to illustrate some of the contrasting elements that are present, even though some patients may appear to share the common feature of talking openly. Susan's ability to cry (overtly showing vulnerability) matched up with the sadness and grief that was expected for a person in her situation. In contrast, Jane's attempts put up a brave front by smiling and telling others not to worry was perceived as behaviour not expected of a person in her situation. Her behaviour appeared incongruent with her ongoing losses and deterioration. It would appear that congruencies and incongruencies between public expressions of emotion and the situations of patients have an important effect on the way particular situations are constructed and defined by nurses.

Other ways of protecting self involved not talking openly about feelings as a means of not being reminded of morbid issues. Often, this involved engaging in superficial talk that was perceived as safe in order to avoid getting too involved, particularly with the other patients in the hospice. This enabled an amount of emotional distance to be maintained. Nonetheless, on occasions this barrier was not invincible. Although attempts were made by patients to protect themselves in this way, the death of others served as a reminder of personal mortality. Those who consciously adopted this strategy were not only upset but became determined to remain uninvolved.

Margaret's approach was to not dwell on morbid matters. She conducted her conversations with the nurses on a surface level, avoiding any cues or leads on issues that appeared to be a threat. Whenever conversations appeared to get close to issues relating to dying, Margaret would close the conversation. This manner of coping was respected by the nurses. Margaret preferred not to talk about the possibility of death or dying and adopted a positive approach. She was happy to talk to me about most things, including reasons for not talking about morbid matters. The following is an extract from a conversation about how she managed her situation.

Case 7 (Margaret)

GC: Margaret, sometimes when people are facing an illness, in terms of going through what you are going through, they like to talk about preparations for their funeral.

M: No, I don't want to know about things like that.

GC: Is it true to say you are not that kind of a person?

M: Yeah, that's true, I'm not. I don't like that sort of thing. I find it morbid.

GC: You find it morbid?

M: Yes, very much so.

GC: You'd rather...

M: I'd rather think about something brighter, gayer. I prefer to look at what's happening now and concentrate on what happened today.

In another conversation we focused on her experiences of coping with the deaths of some of the patients she knew from the hospice.

Case 7 (Margaret)

GC: Recently — and I'm being very open and you can stop me, Margaret — you know there's been a spate of people who have died and it is very sad. Can you tell me how you feel about it?

M: Well, we found it very, very sad. I mean, we got so attached to them, that... and then, I had a good talk to myself and told myself not to get too attached in the future.

GC: How are you going to handle that?

M: I'm going to handle it.

GC: What in particular, makes you very sad?

M: Well, because you got to know them so well. I mean they were here one day and the next day we came they had gone, but I've got over it.

GC: Does it make you think of where you are at, as well, when something like that happens? I mean, does it make you feel that life is very vulnerable for yourself as well, when that happens? Does it remind you of that?

M   No, no, no. I just carry on. You've got to sort of look forward, haven't you? You haven't got to think back, because I love coming here so much and I know it does us all good, and I had an examination the other day. It was quite by chance with the lady doctor and she said that everything is fine. She can't get over how well I am, and she says, that doctor, always says to her I'm a miracle. I am telling you the truth now.

GC: Do you feel cheered up by that?

M: Yes.

Although Margaret tried not to get too attached, six months after this conversation a patient whom she knew died. This had a tremendous impact on her. When she was told about the patient's death, Margaret sobbed with grief.

Unlike Margaret, Sheila (case 8) spoke openly about death and dying and declared that she was not afraid. She said that she welcomed the thought of death when she heard that she had incurable cancer. This view changed in time, resulting in similar strategies used by Margaret (case 7) to protect self. Unlike Margaret who, although divorced, still kept in touch with her family, Sheila, who was also a divorcee, lived on her own and was not in contact with her family. Through using the day centre in the hospice, Sheila became exposed to company, friendship and support. However, it also exposed her to experiences that were sad, such as the death of some of the patients she knew. This experience was particularly upsetting and also threatening for Sheila.

Case 8 (Sheila)

GC: Can you tell me how you're feeling?

S: Since coming as an in-patient for five and a half weeks I'm scared to death of the process of dying. This is one thing that has changed since I last talked to you — I've always accepted death and welcomed it — so lonely and nobody needed me.

GC: What has brought about this change?

S: It was through listening to people dying, crying in pain, people I've spoken to that day, not being there any more, and it upset me terribly.

GC: When you see these things happening do they serve to remind you of one's mortality?

S: Yes, it felt like losing a relation, there's no way I could be dispassionate about it — I cared too much for them as people. I know I've got terminal cancer, no way I could be reminded of that day and night, I couldn't accept that. In fact, if I do wake up, I'm normally screaming. It didn't worry me before but you get to know people, they become real people, you're too frightened to ask what's happened to them.

GC: Do the nurses tell you what's happened to them?

S: Oh yes, they don't hide that from you. Certainly Debbie tells you. I've got a dread of this hospice now. I'm happy as a day centre patient but not as an in-patient. I like the people, also I know I'm going home. I'm scared that I'll die screaming and shouting. I wonder what's ahead of me. I don't seem to be able to take it.

Sheila, like Margaret (case 7), decided not to become too involved with the other patients and in the subsequent months reasserted control by personally reducing her day centre attendance to one day a week instead of the two offered. She also organised to attend a local day centre for people with chronic illness once a week, in addition to her attendance at the hospice.

The extracts from the above case studies (cases 7 and 8) showed how some patients may protect themselves by either choosing to engage through talking openly, or not openly, with others about their situation. The depth of conversation was also significant in 'protecting self' and was often controlled by patients. Exposure to the deaths of others caused sadness and anxiety, even for the patients who may profess no fear of death and dying. Strategies for protecting self in this case involved distancing, by not becoming too attached or involved with others.

The nurses, too, appeared to protect themselves either consciously or unconsciously. Aspects of nurses' protection of self appeared to operate on a daily basis. Often this involved the nurse and patient in conflicting incidents within the course of everyday activities. This interplay of control and protection struck an uneasy balance in certain situations. For instance, Sheila (case 8) appeared to protect herself by preventing nurses and other staff from being too close to her. The need to control situations, combined with a strong sense of independence in the face of progressive losses, made it difficult for Sheila to accept help and for nurses to help Sheila. It became very much a game, where options of care, suggested by nurses and agreed by Sheila, would invariably be turned down by her at the last minute. Moreover, Sheila was sometimes rude about the nurses and doctors and prone to manipulating staff. Despite this, the nurses continued to approach Sheila, even in the most testing circumstances. In conversations with the nurses who had been at the receiving end of some of her rejections, it was particularly revealing how they managed to protect themselves.

Case 8 (Laura: Sheila's nurse)

L: I think that Sheila needs a lot of support and someone needs to be there, however much she tries to push you away. But I think she really needs you there in the end. She's got into the habit of pushing people away.

GC: How do you think she pushes people away?

L: Partly by telling people different stories and manipulating. Perhaps talking behind your back about what you said, you get something completely different.

GC: How do you cope with that?

L: I know that she does it to other people and I know that it's part of her pattern. It tends to be a bit hurtful but I know it's just her and so have to accept that.

GC: Has she ever been angry with you?

L: She was once.

GC: What did she say?

L: She said 'Have you got a pea inside your brain?'. She was the first person I'd ever really been annoyed with, I think, as a patient. And I said: 'Be quiet, Sheila!' and walked out. When I came back later I was completely friendly with her because I felt she needed just checking because I thought that was rather rude.

GC: What did she say to you about you walking away?

L: It wasn't talked about at all.

GC: Why do you think she reacted like that?

L: I think she was quite justified because I had asked her once what the name of her doctor was and then I had to go back and ask her again. So she didn't like me asking her twice.

GC: How did you deal with that feeling of her being angry with you? How did you resolve that within yourself?

L: I wasn't particularly happy about going back anyway to ask her twice, because I felt rather stupid to do it. But I wanted to get it right and so it was partly justified, but I don't think she should have been rude.

GC: How did you deal with a patient being rude to you? Although you went back and talked to her subsequently and were nice to her, what did you do with that at the end of the day?

L: I talked to somebody else about it and we laughed about it.

GC: So that helped?

L: Yes. In my reflective diary I wrote about how I had suggested many different things to try and help her and make her life easier, but she turned down so many things and I felt rather a failure. Although I do know how she behaves with other people, so I can accept it. I did mention that, knowing she has this feeling about not wanting to talk about her family at all, I did mention to her that I was divorced, to perhaps make her feel that other people could feel too.

Other nurses too were at the receiving end of this rejection. The extract below shows how another nurse coped with derogatory remarks.

Case 8 (Kevin: Sheila's nurse)

GC: Do you find her a challenge? Is she difficult to care for?

K: In some respects simply going to her can be difficult in that you find something that's easier to do and you might do that in preference. I certainly found it difficult at the weekend because I overheard her. She was in the smoking room and I was in the kitchen next door. I overheard her talking about me and her perception. What she was saying was quite derogatory. So after that it was even more difficult to get to her because I felt on the one hand I could see things on an intellectual level and think: Well, fine that's me, that's how I am. On a 'feeling' level, it obviously made the threshold quite a lot harder to cross. But on the other hand, I find her by no means the most difficult person I've had to look after or nurse. I don't find approaching her impossible. I think sometimes a person can be far more emotionally draining in the sense that you feel compelled to give more to them because of their need. Whereas with Sheila I don't. The difficulties are only really in a sort of basic relationship and I don't feel any particular compulsion to give very much of myself to her. So in that respect I don't find her particularly demanding. The rest of it — saying inconsistent things or derogatory things about other people or other departments — I can let that roll off my back. I just listen and absorb it at some level and it doesn't really make it particularly hard. I think there may be other people who find that more difficult.

GC: People in your team, you mean?

K: Possibly, but also once or twice people from other teams have sort of come to me and reported things they've overheard Sheila saying, detrimental to other departments, or the ward, whatever. In fact, when you've looked after Sheila for some time you realise and get to know her, or the little you can get to know because there is an awful lot in a sense that's hidden.

GC: Any positive things in terms of caring for people like Sheila (or anybody) that you can actually learn?

K: Yes. Positive things on a neutral level. There is much to be learnt — how to relate to people, looking at the effect they have on us and, to some extent, the effect we have on them, partly reflected by the things that I overheard her saying about me. There is, I suppose, in a strange sort of way satisfaction in doing your best for somebody, however receptive they are or not to that, and doing so regardless of how much you are accepted or rejected.

For these two nurses, reflecting on the incidents, although difficult, helped to construct an internal working framework of managing rejection. For instance, knowing that rejection from that particular patient was not focused solely on them but was also extended to other carers appeared to help in preserving their integrity. Also, holding the view that there was satisfaction to be gained from the work, regardless of acceptance or rejection, may have provided meaning and understanding about the essence of nursing work with dying patients. This may have helped in the continued efforts to approach the patient. By incorporating this construction of meaning within rejection the integrity of the individual nurse appeared intact and protected.

The nurses in the present study did not appear to differ vastly in the approach they adopted to protect themselves when compared with findings of other studies of nurses in similar settings. Personal coping strategies, together with the support system inherent in the hospice, also served as protective mechanisms. Organisationally, there were formal support groups for staff, as well as key people, such as colleagues and counsellors, available to provide support. The hospice culture on the whole cultivates an environment where it is permissible to express feelings and emotions. None of the nurses in the study reported being unsupported (except through the nurse's own choice) in times of sadness, or in situations when it was known that a particular nurse had experienced an emotionally difficult shift.

Summary

The everyday activities of patients who face impending death and the nurses who care for them are complex experiences that involve the acts of protecting and controlling. Patients use talk, either talking openly or not openly about their situations, as part of the process of control, to protect kin, nurses and self. The work of worry serves as a channel for expressing fears and concerns either publicly or privately.

Throughout the course of being a dying patient, the people in this study appeared to juggle with aspects of both public and private fronts. The public front related to the presentation of self to others. The private front was more complex and occurred at several levels, depending on the personality and circumstances of the person and his/her family. This related to personal thoughts and feelings about the disease process, dying and death. Much of this information was relayed to the nurses and, for a few patients, these private accounts were also shared with other patients with whom they had developed a close relationship. The public and private fronts coexisted in harmony on the surface but, on occasions, made for an uneasy partnership at a deeper level. For instance, when the public and private fronts of patients were seen to be at odds — such as when deterioration occurred and further losses were incurred — this appeared problematic, particularly for the nurses. Sometimes tensions arose in the care of patients when there was a perceived mismatch between what was publicly expressed and privately felt. In such situations two main strategies were used by nurses: to regain equilibrium of control by breaking the tension or to let matters take their own course, with the patient in control, until a point was reached when the patient's public and private feelings synchronised.

Various strategies were, nevertheless, tested and used by patients (and nurses) to cope with ongoing losses. These included 'positive' and 'negative' elements of strategic ploys, used primarily as a means to preserve relationships. Castles and Murray (1979, p.101), in their attempts to 'normalise' dying individuals, pointed out some of the negative aspects of human nature that continue as part of being human, despite dying. The authors noted that the dying person uses strategies that 'may strive to control and manipulate the persons around them, so as to prevent significant others from leaving or withdrawing love, or they may pretend to avoid feelings of loss and despair'. Similarly, it was not uncommon to find both positive and negative strategies being used by nurses who care for dying patients as shown by Quint (1967), Melia (1987) and Lichter (1987). My study illustrates further how this interplay of strategies was being acted and managed by individuals within the context of 'taking each day as it comes'.

Nurses also appeared to protect patients and their kin, as well as self. Skilful strategies were used for this, with the nurses often acting as go-betweens for patients, relatives and colleagues. In general, most nurses found patients who talked openly less difficult to care for than those who did not. Balancing the needs of patients and relatives was perceived as a delicate operation. On occasions, some nurses found this act difficult to sustain, particularly when either the spouse or close family members expressed the need for open talking when the patient appeared not ready for it. In these circumstances, emotional support from nurses tended to be shifted towards the needs of the spouse or family members, who were seen as requiring more support. Protecting patients occurred as their physical deterioration progressed. It was carried out as part of control in preventing and overcoming embarrassment. The acts of covering up and pacing were used. Although much of this interplay of protecting and controlling was subsumed under the apparent motivation of concern for another, some of these activities were an indirect means of self-protection.

7. "Past my sell-by date"

Protecting and controlling featured continually throughout the patient's dying trajectory within the routines of 'taking each day as it comes'. However, the patients (and nurses) in this study also had to contend with the issues of time and duration in relation to illness. It was not uncommon for patients to comment on the relationship between duration and the form of their illness — often expressed metaphorically as: 'I'm past my sell-by date'. For some patients, their doctor's original indications about length of survival continued to act as a frame of reference for 'what should be' (that is, I should have died by now according to my doctor) and 'what is' (I'm still alive) and consequently: 'I wonder how much longer I have got?' (I'm out-living my given time or I'm past my sell-by date).

Together with this frame of reference about time, other markers were also used as indicators of disease progression — for instance, the presence or absence of physical deterioration and, invariably, the responses of nurses, doctors and others to their condition. The repertoire of medical treatment offered, such as radiotherapy, chemotherapy and medications to alleviate nausea, vomiting, and pain also acted as cues regarding time. The patients' condition evoked varying responses, some of which were viewed by the patients as positive, and others as negative. The responses mostly concerned how other people reacted to losses associated with the patients' dying and death. In turn, how patients managed these responses and their progressive losses appeared significant in how they constructed meanings from their situations and life.

As losses continued with disease progression the grief expressed by patients became increasingly more apparent and frequent. For most of these patients, deterioration occurred progressively and, apart from periods of remission, the anticipation of the future, in terms of more time for living, was followed by a further increase in physical incapacity and suffering.

Several key patterns were generated during this period of the patients' experience. These were physical fading, which involved bodily deterioration and functioning, social fading, which included planned and unplanned withdrawing from friends and family, and personal fading, which incorporated two facets: a negation of the individual by others and the patient's contemplation of personal mortality. All three patterns intertwined and comprised a mosaic often experienced simultaneously by the patient.

Central to this period of time was the act of watching; patients watched other patients and the nurses, and nurses watched patients (and their families). This was done in tandem with waiting. By watching and waiting for signs and signals, both within and outside of the body, patients and nurses appeared to cue in on physical conditions expressed through the work of 'worry'. This was then lived out by the patient and the nurse through the process of experiencing — feeling and seeing the impact of disease progression against time.

'Watching' was used to construct a picture of disease progression on bodily functions. It was performed inwardly and outwardly. In the former, the focus of watching was on the self (that is, patient-on-self watching) whereas in the latter, other individuals were being watched — patient-on-patient watching or patient-on-nurse watching. Signs of improvement, deterioration or stabilisation were being watched by the patient. In the case of patient-on-nurse watching, clues for the ways professionals perceived the patient's condition and progress were looked for. This information was then used as a frame of reference to judge the process of dying for that individual patient. Similarly, the act of watching was used by nurses, as in nurse-on-patient (and family) and nurse-on-nurse observations.

Numerous accounts of concerns about bodily deterioration were raised during my conversations with patients and nurses. For some patients the period of physical fading was punctuated by periods of stability, where the disease and symptoms appeared to be on hold. For most patients, this stabilisation gradually changed to a path of eventual decline. For a few, however, the stabilisation became long-term remission, and three patients in the study (cases 4, 7 and 8) have continued in remission. While sharing many of the experiences of the other patients in the study, these three have presented alternatives to the theoretical construction of dying roles. Unlike the other patients, whose death was certain (but at an uncertain time), for these three the notion of certain death has become less clear. The interesting and unusual issues raised by these three cases are discussed later in this section.

Nonetheless, in all the cases, watching and waiting for signs and signals from within and outside the body was continuously used by patients and nurses to gauge the extent of the patients' physical condition. Some patients judged their condition by using their external body appearance as a measure. This included weight loss (and weight gain, a side-effect of steroid therapy) and physical functions, such as energy, mobility and continence. Loss of weight, unsurprisingly, appeared to be a major external indicator of physical deterioration. For example, patients such as Carol (case 2) used weight loss to gauge their ability to withstand the progression of their disease by comparing their condition with others. Carol often remarked on her physical decline and compared her own condition with Jane's (case 3):

Case 2 (Carol)

C: I wonder how long it will last, yes I do. I have seen Jane linger for so long and I don't want to be in that state and last a long time. At the moment I can move around and she couldn't. So I don't know how long. I look at myself and how much weight I've lost and I think 'you can't lose much more'.

GC: How much have you lost?

C: I've lost a couple of stones. I wasn't overweight before, so I only weigh about seven stone something. All my clothes are baggy.

GC: Your face is still the same?

C: My face hasn't lost anything, which is surprising really, but my arms, my thighs, my hips…

Just as Carol watched others and herself, she was in turn watched by the nurses as she steadily lost weight. Her nurse commented:

Case 2 (Debbie: Carol's nurse)

GC: Looking at her, do you think there's been a dramatic change?

D: It's been slow but if you haven't seen her for some time you would see quite a difference. She's lost a tremendous amount of weight. She's very fragile-looking and once she hasn't got her make-up on she looks really poorly. She tries so desperately to be the glamorous lady and she is still maintaining that. She had her hair done and her make-up on when she came in yesterday and looked lovely. She's got beautiful pyjamas on and she looked gorgeous. She's beautifully groomed, immaculate, except her clothes are hanging on her a bit now, because she is slowly fading right under your eyes.

Carol's physical decline continued as a very slow process. Although she did not talk openly about her dying it was clear that, privately, physical changes continued to serve as indicators of her own mortality. The extract below shows how, from the nurse's perspective Carol managed and accommodated these physical indicators.

Case 2 (Tina: Carol's nurse)

T: I think that I recognise and respect that Carol doesn't want to talk about death. She has shared with me about the death of her husband. But as far as her own death and dying are concerned she is just not prepared to talk about it, although it is quite clear she knows she is dying. Yesterday we actually discussed the skin changes she had undergone and she accepted that this was the cancer spreading. She looked quite deep in thought and appeared to be thinking deeply about it and knew that there was nothing she could do, or I could do, to change things. So she's just plodding on, really.

Carol's fragile condition appeared to evoke feelings of protectiveness from some of the nurses, who worried about her struggling at home, despite Carol's choice to do so. Carol continued in this slow decline until, eventually, a fall at home resulted in her admission and subsequent death.

Signs and signals from within the body were also watched for by patients and nurses. Unlike external indicators, which can be more immediately seen, these internal physical indicators were 'felt or experienced' by patients. For instance, the development of a new pain in a different part of the body can only be experienced by the patient and, unless expressed, may not be obvious to others. The development of new signs and symptoms was normally followed by waiting for confirmation of disease progression as a result of investigations such as X-rays, scans and blood tests.

The progressive onset of disease was particularly distressing for Susan (case 1). As she deteriorated, unlike Carol (case 2), Susan's weight remained constant, although she felt physically unwell.

Case 1 (Susan)

S: Most times, it has been reasonable, but just recently it's got worse because of the pain. I have medication which controls it but then it upsets the stomach and I don't know whether it's the tablets or me. And I climb the stairs and when I get to the top of the stairs, my head just goes boom, boom boom, you know, and I have to stand there for a few minutes before I do anything. Any exertion, it's just hopeless. I can't even change the sheets on the bed now. I'm okay if I'm sitting, I can sew or read. If I'm sitting and doing nothing, I'm fine, but as I say, I've tried to change the beds or collect the washing-up to put in the washer, and my head goes boom, boom, boom and I just have to sit. I can do about 10 minutes then I sit and then I do a bit more. I never know when the next pain is going to start. Saturday it was just my arm aching, because of the radiotherapy, Sunday, it was a stabbing pain in my back rib, you know it just comes so quickly and suddenly, and I'm just frightened that something might happen.

In a later interview, as Susan continued to deteriorate, there were indications that her predicament was confounded by peoples' perception of her and her desire to put on a brave face. Because she looked well, there was an assumption that she was fine.

S: I really try to forget about things and carry on as normal, because everybody says: 'You look so well'. I don't think my father understands. I'm sure he doesn't. I only came out of hospital on Wednesday and he came yesterday and I made a big meal last night. I just felt exhausted afterwards. I think he just thinks that I'm managing very well. I suppose I am. I put on a brave face, that's what it is.

As Susan continued to deteriorate, she found it increasingly difficult to carry on with activities such as ironing, gardening and going for walks. Blood tests showed low haemoglobin and platelet counts. There were also considerable liver and bony metastases. Susan continued to feel tired, breathless and weak. In the following conversation, she talked about her future, watching the progression of her physical condition.

GC: How have you been, Susan?

S: At the moment, I don't know. I am very confused because I've had more bad news.

GC: What was the bad news?

S: The cancer has gone into my bone marrow. It's a progression of the illness. I just don't know how long it can keep me going like this. I had a transfusion six weeks ago and it didn't really last six weeks. By the end of the fifth week I started to feel ill again. So I had some more blood, more transfusions but not as many. I had five units last time, this time I had four units. But I don't feel as well as after I had the first one. I'm fine just sitting, doing nothing, but as soon as I start to move around or bend or do anything, I'm just weak.

GC: Have you had time to reflect a bit more on what's happening? How does that leave you?

S: To be quite honest, I feel now that I'm not going to be here this time next year. I sort of think of things and I think, well, I'll probably not be here. I don't know, nobody knows, do they, but I just feel because I know what my body is telling me.

Just as patients appeared to watch the impact of disease progression on their bodies, nurses too watched the patients and waited to see the impact of treatments. This seemed to enable nurses to construct a picture of the patient's physical condition and define their dying status. Constant references to internal disease spread were made to provide a reference point with regard to time, duration and shape of the disease and its course. For instance, when asked whether she perceived Susan's condition to be deteriorating, her nurse responded:

Case 1 (Debbie: Susan's nurse)

D: I think so. There is quite a lot of liver involvement. It's quite big, the liver, and I know she's got some more cord compression, and her blood is not staying up, it's gone right back down again. She's had blood transfusions now, three to four weeks. The whole situation is deteriorating dramatically. I thought she was dying three months ago. I wouldn't have thought she would have gone on much longer with the deterioration that's happening.

Susan continued to deteriorate and chose to carry on with blood transfusions until the time of her death.

As patients entered this 'past my sell-by date' period, the combination of physical deterioration, with treatments and investigations, became more prominent than before. Physically, more time was taken up with treatments and symptom control. For some, treatments such as radiotherapy, chemotherapy, steroid therapy and blood transfusions were offered as part of the palliative regimes to control the spread of disease, alleviate pain and increase a sense of well-being. Such treatments continued to provide a measured amount of quality of life by containing further deterioration. In other words, without the treatments, physical decline and disease spread were likely to be more rapid. Although treatments enabled some patients to 'buy' a reasonable quality of life, there were also trade-offs. Watching the impact of these treatments on their bodies, coping with the side-effects and waiting for and then experiencing the benefits of treatment were matters of concern frequently expressed by the patients (and their nurses). Moreover, the pacing of doctor's appointments and treatments was watched and provided signs for gauging the impact of the treatment on the progression of the disease.

Lyn (case 5), continued with a reasonable quality of life for over a year, sustained by a series of treatments that included chemotherapy, steroid and hormonal therapy and drainage of a pericardial effusion. Lyn talked openly about her condition and, like Jane (case 3), maintained a cheerful public front most of the time. The impact of the treatments and the sense of living on borrowed time are vividly described in the following accounts of her experiences. Below is an extract of how Lyn watched the pacing of appointments in order to construct an understanding of the course of her disease against the effects of treatments.

Case 5 (Lyn)

GC: Lyn, we were talking just now, and you told me that the doctors don't need to see you for another two months and you always go by that. Tell me a bit about that.

L: Oh dear [laughs]. Well, I know. I had cancer before; they start off by seeing you every three weeks or every month and then they go to seeing you every two months or three months and then it goes to every six months and then it goes to a year. So I know by that they think you are doing well if they keep on seeing you the same amount of time, or a shorter amount of time if they are worried about you.

GC: So that gives you an indicator?

L: Yes, it gives you a bit of confidence, really, that you are feeling quite well.

GC: So have you any more thoughts about the disease itself?

L: I just get on with it [life] and I don't think much about it [disease]. I get a bit out of breath, but that's all. But no, I just carry on ordinary. I don't do anything different and I don't think: I can't do this and I can't do that. I get moaned at for picking up everything [laughs]. I can pick up the heavy things, I just do what I can do, I can do everything now that I was doing before and the doctors are pleased with that. The only thing I don't do is work. But I cut the grass with a handmower, a push handmower, and I ride my bike everywhere. Except, I don't ride up such big hills now. So I do everything the same.

GC: So you're pleased with that?

L: Yes. I'm very pleased with that because I couldn't first of all. I've gradually got stronger.

Lyn's positive attitude to life enabled her to cope with many of the external changes that she experienced as a result of the treatments she underwent. For instance, during the time that she was bald due to chemotherapy she wore a wig, washed and pegged it on the washing line and used it as a talking point about her cancer with her neighbour, thus breaking down a conventionally taboo subject in conversations. She gained weight and, despite a puffy, round and fully stretched face (side-effects of steroid therapy), Lyn bore the additional discomfort with fortitude because of the additional quality time that the drugs would give her. The account below indicates how she felt when her physical condition began to change, when a critical point was reached at which treatments and drug therapy were unable to contain her disease.

GC: What sort of drugs are you on now, Lyn?

L: Quite low, but I'm back on chemo.

GC: Your face, it's now more puffy?

L: Steroids, loads of steroids.

GC: So when did that happen?

L: My liver started going, too bad.

GC: What do you mean by that?

L: Although my cancer attacks my heart, I have also got it in my lungs and my liver and my lymph glands and my bones, and they thought my liver, I don't understand what it is, but I think they thought it was crystallising or something, so they put me on loads of steroids, so within five weeks my face has come up like a balloon.

GC: This is why it's a bit rounder.

L: If I go anymore I won't see out of my eyes.

GC: Does that bother you?

L: Not too much, it just feels a bit uncomfortable, because it's hard, it's very hard under your chin. But for five weeks to come up and you feel like when you put your hands on your cheeks, you feel like they're a few feet away. But the steroids make you feel an awful lot better, because two months ago I really felt like I was really going downhill. I was going downhill so fast that I didn't think I would live a lot longer.

GC :   When they talk about the cancer going into your liver, and all that, does that make you think that things are not working out as well as you expected?

L: Well, I am living longer than what they said I would live, and past my sell-by date, as I say. I had it in my liver last year, and although I didn't have it in my lungs last year, when I had this cardiac done, this time it was the same cardiac doctor, that I always have, and he was asking me about my cancer and he said: 'You didn't have it in your lungs' and he thought last year I had it in my lungs. So when they told me a week later it had gone to my lungs I was prepared for it, because this doctor had actually said he thought it was already in my lungs and my liver. I had it in my liver last year and they cured it, but it is back again, so it wasn't too much of a surprise. It must be weaker.

GC: You mentioned you're past your sell-by date. Does that mean you do things differently now? How do you look at life?

L: I don't. I just carry on as normal. I can't do it any other way. Some people say they like to change their life completely, whereas I don't. I just carry on as normal as I can. I still moan at my friend sometimes!

Lyn continued with her chemotherapy and treatments until the time of her death. She was seen by the oncologist, who eventually told her that chemotherapy would no longer be useful as part of her overall treatment package. I asked Lyn how she took that news. She said that she felt alright because she did not want any more chemotherapy. Moreover, during this appointment with the doctor she was taken to a room which she called the 'bad news room'. By that time, according to her, she was already prepared for what they were going to say.

As deterioration continued, a critical juncture was reached by most patients when it became clear to everyone that their body was beginning to shut down and could no longer benefit from, or tolerate, further treatments. At this point, the patient was perceived to enter the terminal phase.

However, in contrast to the cases highlighted above, the physical condition of three patients (cases 4, 7 and 8) continued to plateau and gave the impression of being on long-term hold. The dying trajectories of these three patients therefore shifted from 'certain death at an unknown time' to a 'suspended-sentence trajectory' (Glaser and Strauss, 1968). For these three patients the disease and symptoms were in remission and long periods of time elapsed in which there was no further significant deterioration. This change in the construction of an expected dying trajectory created a degree of uncertainty for the patients and the nurses. For instance, patients and nurses indicated having to redefine and reconstruct the meaning of the dying role, which hitherto had been a key transitional phase for the patients to accommodate, and for the nurses to prepare and facilitate as the patients entered hospice care. A focal point of tension centred on what was a suitable place of long-term care for these surviving individuals. The feelings of unease, guilt and tension that arose over this issue, particularly for the nurses, are described in detail in Chapter 9. As the threat of impending death decreased for the three surviving patients, both mundane and exceptional everyday life activities became increasingly significant. These issues are illustrated below in the selected extracts from cases 4 and 7.

Case 4 (Ian)

GC: Ian, in terms of where you are with your cancer, I gather that's improved?

I: Yes, my cancer is in remission. It's been five years now, which is good news. We hope it stays that way. I don't have any contact with London [referring to his consultant] now unless something happens.

GC: How do you feel in terms of where you are now, with the future?

I: In the future? I've not really got that far. Being much better I can make arrangements which I never did before. I've been able to plan my holidays now, which I haven't done since the cancer problem started. I'd like to make plans for September to go on holiday for two weeks abroad, which is something I've never dreamt about.

GC: You mean you can be more sure of making plans, future plans like holidays, more so than what you were able to do before?

I: Oh yes, my life is such now that I can have more confidence, I can say that certain dates we can go away and have two weeks' holiday. I find it easier to do now than I did before.

The following two extracts are taken from two separate interviews on Margaret's (case 7) physical condition. The second extract was recorded four months after the first. The interviews show how normal everyday activities had become more significant for Margaret as her disease continued to be in remission.

Case 7 (Margaret)

GC: Margaret, when you became ill, how did your family respond to it? I mean, what were their feelings about it?

M: Well, they were very upset. You know, they thought I wouldn't survive.

GC: How do you feel about this now, surviving?

M: I feel fine, thanks, great. All I've got now is a bit of sciatica but I can put up with that — I had it last year. But in myself I'm great and I'm eating and eating and I can't eat enough now and drink.

GC: How are you feeling now?

M: I am feeling back to my normal self now. I go out more, I go down the town on the bus. I go all over the place now. I am feeling a lot better.

GC: Your hair has also grown.

M: Yes. They said after the chemo it would. They say it always grows thicker and more curly.

GC: What are your plans in terms of the future?

M: Just carry on. Nothing in particular, just enjoy the day. Take it from day to day. I don't over-exhaust myself on anything. I just take it quietly.

GC: How have you found it being in the day centre?

M: I like it. I look forward to it. Two days a week — Tuesday and Thursday — and I like the company. I like the day care, the volunteers and as I said before I can't thank the doctors enough for getting me well.

GC: Looking back now to what you were like before, what is the comparison in terms of what you were like before and now? The differences?

M: I don't think I'm the same as I was before my illness. I was talking about it the other day. Well, I haven't got the energy like I had before, maybe because I am getting older. It could be old age.

GC: You noticed that you've got less energy?

M: Yes, but I feel fine. As I say, I've got a marvellous appetite. I sleep very well all night.

GC: You don't have any of the dreams that you've talked about before?

M: Oh no, that's all gone. I put it down to my illness when I was dehydrated. That wasn't very pleasant. But all that's gone and I have ordinary dreams.

GC: Is there anything else you would like to tell me, anything more significant that has happened in your life?

M: Not really, I'm just content as I am now. I can get my own meals and do my own housework better now. As I say, if I feel like going out I just get on the bus and take it easy. When I'm in town I go and have a Guinness, then do a bit more shopping and get the bus home.

GC: Do you think that's almost like back to being normal again?

M: Yes.

Both Ian's and Margaret's experiences of their remission were confirmed by the same nurse in the extracts below. Nevertheless, there appeared to be a feeling of guilt on the nurse's behalf for encouraging the patients to be more accepting of their situation. It also appeared that, with a disease such as cancer, despite the patients' feelings of being well and evidence of remission there remained a constant fear that the disease may relapse.

Case 4 (Laura: Ian's nurse)

GC: Ian was diagnosed to have quite an aggressive teratoma and it was thought that he was dying, with secondaries. And now suddenly it seems we are going the other way in terms of trying to get him to move out of his dying role. How do you cope with that?

L: Well, I feel a little bit guilty that is the course I have encouraged because that's how I saw my role to help to be more accepting of how he was. But now that he is better I think you do have to think about encouraging him to do more for himself.

GC: How does Ian feel about this ?

L: When I actually suggested to him about going to the rehabilitation unit for perhaps one day a week he did seem quite... He said: 'I feel as though I have got in a rut' and he did seem quite enthusiastic about it. Since then I have tried to encourage him at the day centre to do a few things. I just asked him what he would like to do. Perhaps if he would like to do cooking because he used to be a baker or he suggested he would like to do woodwork, because that's something he always wanted to do. But then when I said should we start it now he said: 'Well, I think.' He always put it off and then in the end he did actually decide he would make a plastic basket.

GC: Does he see himself as being cured? Do you have a feeling in terms of how he views his illness?

L: I think when we have been trying to reduce his visits to London for his check-ups there has been terrific anxiety by his wife that she wants him still to be checked up and doesn't want to let go. It seems very hard for them. To be quite honest, I feel quite nervous of addressing the fact, of saying you're cured, because I feel it's such an unsure thing, how can we really say that? I think the reason is, it is such a big issue for someone to perceive themselves as perhaps dying and then for anybody to put the idea into their head that they are not and maybe later on they will be dying at some stage. But to be sure of that is a very difficult thing to say to anybody.

Case 7 (Laura: Margaret's nurse)

GC: What are your feelings about caring for her as a nurse. Do you find it challenging? How would you describe it?

L: I do feel a little bit worried if she were to have the cancer come back again because I think she would be absolutely devastated. She has put all her trust now in being well again. I asked her today if she was thinking about going on holiday and she said she had had such a terrible shock last time she went on holiday [she became ill] that she's very frightened to actually go again.

Although Sheila's account has not been presented here, a similar pattern was observed and Sheila gained more confidence and continued to carry on with her life, attending the day centre once a week.

In most cases, social and personal fading was observed to occur as physical deterioration progressed. Social fading refers to a situation where, as the patient's physical abilities and functions progressively decline, the ability to be sociable — holding conversations and participating in everyday activities — becomes increasingly difficult. This is marked by a process of gradual physical and mental withdrawal, which appears eventually to modify some of the sociable characteristics of the person's make-up.

For instance, increasing weakness and fatigue were observed to occur in conjunction with bouts of nausea, vomiting, and pain, which progressively limited the ability of some of the patients to pursue interests and interact with others. To an extent, the course of physical deterioration was dependent on the type of cancer. Cancers such as cerebral tumours affect the neurological functioning of the body and limit mobility, speech and memory (Obbens, 1993). Patients deteriorating with tumours of this type became severely hampered in their ability to socialise. It was painful to watch this process, which had profound effects on other patients, staff, family and friends. Often social contacts with friends and neighbours became situations of unease, in which discussions about the health and condition of the dying person was avoided. This seemed to be a contributory factor to personal fading, creating a situation in which the personal self of the individual was negated.

Personal fading refers to a process that is inextricably linked to social and physical fading. It may be experienced as a consequence of an insidious process of subtle social rejection and shunning of the dying brought about partly by having incurable cancer and presenting an external appearance associated with bodily deterioration. These social experiences appeared to be particularly met outside the hospice setting.

Personal fading may also be experienced through the patients' personal constructions of future events in relation to redefinitions of self and time. During the period of 'past my sell-by date' some patients began contemplating their own demise — for instance, talking about future events that included them yet, at the same time, acknowledging that they may not be part of that future event. This contemplation of non-being appeared particularly difficult for young patients with growing families who felt there was still much to live for.

From my conversations with the patients, there were numerous accounts of their observations and experiences of social and personal fading as direct and indirect consequences of their body deterioration. A few are presented below.

Case 1 (Susan)

S: My friends, I have had support from them, but unfortunately during the time that I've had the breast cancer some of my friends have moved away, which has upset me because it has left me quite lonely. They still keep in touch with me, but what I find harder is neighbours who, although they weren't what I would call close friends, I realise they can't cope with it, and I never see them. They never come round and ask how I am. There were about three that I was quite friendly with, and Anne... we asked a few people in at Christmas for a drink, she never even asked how I was, and I think that she probably can't cope with it, but I find that quite hard. And another neighbour who, before I was taken ill, all she did was talk about her health, she thought that she had a bad heart and used to go on and on about this heart trouble. Occasionally I see her and she never even mentions it. I just find that so hard.

Case 4 (Ian)

GC: You were saying how people respond to you?

I: Yes, they feel embarrassed. Well, that's the impression I get from a lot of people. They feel uncomfortable in my presence.

GC: How does that feel, for you?

I: In the beginning it made me a bit angry because I thought, well, I've not changed. I couldn't see any difference in me as a person. Alright, I've got cancer but, I thought, what difference does that make? A lot of people gave me the impression that they were afraid. They were sorry for me, then they were afraid to get too close to me — people I've known for years. All of a sudden there was this sort of barrier drawn just like that. That did make me angry. I used to think: well, why? Why do they do that? They gave me the impression that they were embarrassed when I was about. A lot of people couldn't look at me. If they were in the room with me they would look everywhere rather than look where I was. I got the feeling of embarrassment on their side, not mine, because I'm not embarrassed about it. As I said, it made me angry at first. After a time I thought, well, the reality is they couldn't cope with it, they couldn't handle it. They knew me when I was well, but now I am ill they think I'm different, but I'm not really. To yourself and your personality it shouldn't make any difference whether you're ill or well. For a long time this puzzled me. I even asked my wife, but she didn't know. She told me not to worry about them, that's her policy.

Together with having to endure discrimination because of his illness, Ian also had to cope with the discrediting manner in which people behaved towards him when he used his wheelchair. He felt that his dignity and self-esteem (attributes of his personal self) were being continuously diminished by some people as a direct consequence of having an incurable disease and physical disability. Ian went on to say:

I: A lot of people look at you when you are in a wheelchair and think: poor soul — and I think that is unkind. I'm in a wheelchair for only one reason — it is more comfortable and I get less pain. That's the only reason I'm in it. When I'm out and I'm in a wheelchair and we see somebody they don't talk to me, they talk to my wife. Why don't they talk to me? If they are asking a question about me, they ask my wife. I've said to people: 'Look I'm here, you can ask me, I know better than she does.' A lot of people used to say 'How is he today?' I used to think: ask me, I am here and I can tell you exactly how I am feeling. Some people get embarrassed. Some people say they don't know why they ask her and not me. People treat you as if you are an imbecile, incapable of speaking or talking to them and answering their question. My wife is getting into the habit now of when somebody asks her how I am, she'll say: 'Ask him.' This is how she copes with it because she knows how angry it makes me. They treat me as though I wasn't there or in any fit condition to answer them.

Similarly, Alison's case (case 6) illustrates the impact of how a young patient copes with social rejection.

Below are extracts of my conversations with Alison and her nurse, showing their construction of events in this particular incident

Case 6 (Alison)

GC: When you think back, Alison, in terms of how you were, six months ago, do you notice any change in you?

A: Oh yes.

GC: What changes?

A: I'm not having the seizures. The seizures were really difficult to cope with. It's easier for me to live at home, one of the girls I'm still finding it difficult to get on with, but in that respect I'm feeling a lot better. I'm slowly becoming capable of doing jobs in the house and garden. It still takes a long time, I'm aware of that, but I accept that now. It annoys me sometimes, I get upset, but on the whole I can cope with them now.

GC: You mentioned the other girl in the house that you didn't get on so well with. Was it to do with you being ill?

A: Yes, it's to do with me being ill, because she can't accept it. Now, I've accepted it, I've had a year and a half to accept it, but for my friend, she finds it difficult, that I'm not going to the pub any longer, that I'm not being part of that laughing, joking section.

GC: So it's really accepting you as you are?

A: Yes, she finds it difficult. We are still friends but she will only show her friendship when there are other friends within the environment. When it's just her and me in the house she will avoid me, which breaks my heart, and it must be hurting her as well... but I haven't got the courage to speak to her. Maybe that will come, or maybe the friendship is dying. I don't know, you don't know these things.

GC: Makes you wonder why she feels this way?

A: She misses a friend, I should imagine, the same as I miss her friendship.

GC: And the rest of your other friends, are they alright with you?

A: Yes, fine. We have a lot of crying sessions together but that's what it's all about. At least we can talk about it.

Six months after this conversation, the situation deteriorated and Alison was told to get out by Susan, her housemate. This was distressing for Alison and affected those who cared for her, as exemplified by the following account from her nurse, who watched the events unfolding:

Case 6 (Debbie: Alison's nurse)

D: The situation at home had been getting increasingly worse and worse with the tension. It's an ongoing situation. But Susan had actually turned round to Alison and said she doesn't want her to live with her any more. Susan had been her friend for eight years. They've known each other very, very well, but Susan's always found it difficult to accept the illness and the body change of Alison, and Alison's lifestyle as well has altered dramatically. Susan has been isolating Alison in the house for a long time. But in fact, it has now come to a head and Susan has actually asked Alison to move out and doesn't want her to live there any more. When Alison asked her why she said: 'You are not the same, you have changed.'

The nurse felt for Alison, and expressed anger at this treatment of her.

D: Really, we are in the game of finding her alternative accommodation. We have in fact gone down three avenues, the housing department who are looking for accommodation for her, a private person whom we have used here in the past, Jane, who helped us with Anne, who was our other cerebral tumour patient, and in fact, the third avenue was one that Alison has investigated herself. It is a friend of the family who has a house and lets it off in flats and that's been successful, which is super actually, because it is a self-contained flat.

The joy and satisfaction of seeing Alison maintaining her independence and in control of her situation was evident in the way the nurse talked about the outcome of this particular incident. Alison subsequently moved into this flat and lived there with support until she was unable to do so any longer.

In contrast to the above cases, the process of social fading and rejection can also arise as a result of patients' own choice. For instance, a few patients found the journeys to the hospice particularly tiring as they became weaker. Ted (case 9) and Jane (case 3) preferred to be at home, supported by the Macmillan nurse from the hospice and the local primary health care team. In both cases, the patients' social world became increasingly confined to home and to visits from family, close friends and the community health care team. Moreover, there were indications too of withdrawal and rejection towards others who visited at home.

Case 3 (Jane)

GC: Do you feel you've got less energy?

J: Yes. Everything needs a bit of an effort. Like yesterday, a girlfriend I went to school with came with her husband for the day and they went about 5pm. I was really glad to see the back of them. It sounds nasty but I was exhausted really. I was asleep before they got out of the door, and I thought: 'Oh God, I wish they'd leave me alone.' I'm gradually sort of seizing up, but I'm long past my time.

Similarly, in Carol's case (case 2), she chose to remain alone in her home and when she had to be admitted there were also indications of withdrawal as her condition deteriorated. For instance, Carol's withdrawal from people became more evident as she became weaker. Although Carol had never really talked openly about her condition she appeared more detached and noncommunicative. This was particularly so on one of her admissions to the hospice. Carol's haemoglobin level fell to 7.5 g/dl. She declined a blood transfusion and was weak and pale. She spent considerable periods of her time resting in bed, turning down offers by nurses to take her to the day centre to participate in social activities. The only time Carol brightened up was in the evenings when her son Mike visited. The nurses who looked after Carol found her detachment and withdrawal difficult.

Case 2 (Nora: Carol's nurse)

GC: How have you found Carol today or since she has come in?

N: I think generally we feel we are not communicating with her. She is quite withdrawn and has become more detached than when I remember her. I actually find that I can't ask her directly what she is thinking, because I feel that is intrusive and I think she wouldn't want it.

GC: How does this compare with the last time she was in?

N: I met her a year ago when I first started on the ward and she was much more forthright and communicative, talking about going home and how she was going to be cared for at home. I have seen her in the day centre since and she again has been much more communicative and outward-looking. The thing is, at the moment I actually feel she wants to talk but it's just really finding the right time and not being there too long to make the situation embarrassing. I would be interested to know actually how to approach it really.

GC: Why do you think she is like she is at the moment? Any thoughts?

N: I think one thing is she has got pain. She has not got pain when she is lying still but she has pain on movement. I have asked her if she wants more drugs and she doesn't appear to. She doesn't really appear to be any more sleepy but she doesn't want any input from television, books, radio or anything like that. It seems to me she is saving herself up for the evening when she actually gets up in a chair and spends time if someone like her son is here, trying to look as good as possible.

The process of withdrawing and being detached from social activities appeared, to an extent, dependent on the physical condition and character of the person. Although this withdrawal was perceived as a form of rejection by the nurses it also presented an interesting dimension with regard to how patients conserve energy for what may be their most important activities. This was expressed in different ways. For instance, in Jane's case she was conserving her energy for her immediate circle of family and known health carers. In Carol's case, all her energy was conserved in order for it to be directed for a short period of time to her son, who was the person most important to her. Thus, it is crucial that the need for patients to withdraw and conserve what little energy they have left for the most important part of their living is understood by those nursing dying patients in order to provide sensitive care at this critical time.

As well as withdrawing from the social world, it appeared that the process of personal fading was also experienced through the patients' personal constructions of future events. Such critical moments appeared to be instrumental in shaping the person's redefinition of self and time as they watched their deteriorating physical condition. Often, patients would touch on the subject of their 'non-being'.

During our conversations, Susan (case 1) talked about not knowing how long she had left to live, and she would touch tearfully on aspects of family life of which she knew she could not be part. Family events — for instance, her niece's wedding — were emotional times for Susan. The wedding served as a reminder that she would not see her own daughter married and, moreover, that this would be the last occasion when all the 'family members will be together'. The thought of those losses were at times overwhelming for Susan. Below is an account of her thoughts evoked by the event:

Case I (Susan)

S: Tomorrow my sister's daughter is getting married, so we are going to the wedding. My father is coming to stay. He is 82. All the family will be together. I'm frightened I'm going to be a bit tearful.

GC: Would they understand?

S: It's not that. I just feel that I've got a beautiful daughter, not that I want to push her down the aisle or anything like that, but I can't imagine her getting married. I would just love to see her settled. It's silly because she's only 20. I think just the family altogether would probably be the last time.

Implicit in this conversation was an awareness on Susan's part that she may not live and be part of such future occasions. This created a profound sense of loss whenever she allowed herself to glimpse, albeit fleetingly, the situation of her non-being.

Similarly, a few months after he was referred to the hospice, James (case 11) began to deteriorate and expressed profound sadness and grief about his imminent death. He talked openly about his desire to remain alive in order to see the birth of his two grandchildren. The first of these, according to James, had been achieved. Having been told he had only six weeks to live he had survived past that time to see his first grandchild. His next hope was to see his second grandchild. He was also concerned about his wife and family and wondered whether he was 'letting them down'. James expressed openly and sadly between tears that he would 'like to be alive in two years time'. Statements such as 'I'm dying and I really want to be up and dancing with my grandchildren' were openly made.

Considerable grief and sadness were evoked from patients' personal contemplation into their imminent mortality and non-being. Although the examples above show aspects of grief for the loss of self that are related to future losses, there were also examples from patients' conversations demonstrating grief that related to previous as well as current losses.

The course of dying involves both time and form. Of the 12 patients in the study, from the time of referral to the hospice four (cases 1, 10, 11 and 12) survived under a year (range 4-10 months), five (cases 2, 3, 5, 6 and 9) survived one to two years (range 18-24 months), and three patients (cases 4 ,7 and 8) have continue to survive (range 4-7 years). The period of time in which deterioration was manifest, expressed metaphorically by some patients as 'past my sell-by date', appeared as an important phase for the patients and their nurses. Markers appeared to be used by patients to gauge the progression of their disease. These included the acts of watching and waiting. Watching involved observing for physical signs of improvement, deterioration and stabilisation. Watching by patients also took the form of one or more of the following: patient-on-self watching, patient-on-patient/others watching, or patient-on-nurse watching.

Similarly, nurses too seemed to use the act of watching as in nurse-on-patient (and family), or nurse-on-nurse. At the same time as watching, the act of waiting also occurred. This often involved waiting to see what happened or waiting with the patient. Within this, three key patterns have also been identified. They are physical, social and personal fading. All three patterns appeared to be intertwined and may be seen as mosaic in nature, often experienced simultaneously by the patient concerned.

8. "I don't know how to die"

As the patient's body began to shut down physically it became clear to all who continued to watch, wait, protect and control that, despite intensive treatments, the person's body could no longer benefit from or was able to tolerate treatments. This signalled to the patient that death was close. During this period, each patient's experiences and state of readiness to die appeared to vary. The expression 'I don't know how to die' was used by some patients, and it was equally common to find the nurses commenting that a particular patient did not know how to die.

The process of dying or how to die is rarely discussed, despite the certainty that every individual will experience it, except in cases of sudden death. In most other life experiences, such as childbirth or surgery, it is common for the person to tell others about the experience, but this is not so with the process of dying. It is only people alongside the dying person, such as nurses, relatives or other patients, who usually learn about dying. They rarely talk about their experience in view of the perceived morbid nature of the topic, with the result that knowledge about the dying process remains relatively unshared. It is not surprising, therefore, that most people 'don't know how to die'.

This phenomenon is complex and as I followed the patients it became clear that the experience of not knowing how to die arose in combination with several major factors that were critical to them. These included family attachments, the extent of physical incapacity and psychological accommodation to withdraw from the present life. All of these played a part in contributing to the person's state of readiness to die.

HOLDING ON AND LETTING GO

Only a few studies have explored the interactional processes that occur during the terminal phase of dying. Drawing from a few early studies of this phenomenon, Pattison (1977) said that, according to Lieberman (1965), Davis (1973) and Norton (1963), the terminal phase is marked by a gradual turning from the outside world to the internal self. Physical and psychological withdrawal as well as 'emotional disorganisation' have been observed to occur.

In this study, the terminal period of dying appeared more complex than earlier studies have projected. The person's state of readiness to die was shaped by the acts of holding on and letting go, which seemed to be integral components of the process. The acts of holding on and letting go appeared dynamic, staggered and sometimes symmetrical, located on the continuum of the person's dying trajectory. For instance, some patients (cases 1, 5, 9 and 11) continued to hold on to life despite bodies that were in rapid physical decline. They appeared to struggle with dying and their deaths were observed as difficult. Others (cases 2, 3 and 10) were ready, and when their physical condition deteriorated they appeared to die without struggle. Two patients (cases 6 and 12) continued to hold on and let go in a variable manner. While accepting that their deaths were imminent, they periodically resisted by using denial-like mechanisms, depending on whether their physical condition continued to hold out or to decline. However, as their physical condition deteriorated, both patients lapsed into semi-consciousness and died quietly in their sleep. Three patients (cases 4, 7 and 8) continued to hold on in a physically stable condition while their disease remained in remission. In total, seven (cases 1, 2, 5, 6, 10, 11 and 12) patients died in the hospice, one (case 9) died in the local acute general hospital and one died at home (case 3).

Acts of holding on and letting go involved not only patients but also their relatives and nurses, and the overall balance of these processes contributed to the patient's state of readiness to die. Two components were identified as important on the patient's thoughts and wishes about death and their style of dying. Enmeshed within these components were the patient's feelings for others and for self, which might or might not involve a desire to give up the present life. This seemed to depend on the strength of family attachments, projection of a public front and the extent to which life still remained important. The extent to which bodily deterioration and patients' desire to hold on were matched or mismatched affected the degree of anguish, sorrow, tension and conflict experienced by the family, nurses and patient.

During the terminal period patients, relatives and nurses engaged in an intensive phase of watching and waiting for death. The interplays between physical, psychological and social factors appeared increasingly intense within the everyday nurse-patient encounters. For the nurses, too, there were indications of a shift from an initially supportive nursing role to an increasingly combined 'doing for' role for the patient.

As each patient's condition deteriorated, constructions of 'body-person split' in determining their readiness to die became increasingly evident. For instance, some patients talked about their bodies as a separate entity from themselves in relation to the disease process and in preparing for funerals. In contrast, the nurses appeared to separate the patient's physical body from his/her personal self in their talk as death approached. The constructions of a body-person split were made by direct reference to the body as a separate entity from the personal self of the individual.

The following sections present selected accounts of patients' and nurses' constructions of death and dying that illustrate the phenomenon of body-person split as well as patients' individual manner of dying. The latter will incorporate nurses' accounts of the events leading up to the patients' death, or continued survival.

Thoughts of patients and nurses on death and dying

During my conversations with the patients, almost all expressed thoughts and wishes about how they would like their own deaths to be. These expressions were constructed around personal feelings, desires and beliefs about death and dying, often contrasted with observations of dying and death, either through watching family members who had died or the death of patients in the hospice. Observations of how others died seemed to reinforce, and sometimes to have modified, personal views and beliefs about death. Most of the patients expressed a desire for their deaths to occur quickly and wanted to avoid a prolonged death, although this was not always achieved because of the gradual progression of the malignant disease.

Jane (case 3) described herself as an atheist and often talked publicly of her thoughts and wishes about her own death and dying. The first extract was obtained when she was still physically mobile and attending the day centre at the hospice. Here Jane interspersed her views of her own death with a touch of black humour. Throughout her illness, Jane expressed her desire for a quick and peaceful death.

Case 3 (Jane)

GC: Jane, what thoughts go through your mind in terms of your own death?

J: Well, I've got angina and I don't take my angina tablets because I'd rather go with angina than cancer. Having said that, I'm not as brave as I sound because, although I don't take the tablets, on one occasion I was having an angina attack, I thought: 'I'm going to sit through this, I'm not going to take any tablets, and I will die painfully, maybe, but quickly.' In actual fact I ended up gasping 'get my tablets'. The other day I had an angina attack in bed. I felt this attack coming on and I thought: right, I'm really not going to take anything this time. So I got myself all organised, straightened myself in bed, and I was holding Ron's hand and I'd go through this when I suddenly thought 'Oh Lord, if I die I'll get *rigor mortis* and he'd wake up in the morning sort of clasping a dead hand, and shoot through the window with shock.' By the time I got all this organised, the pain was going away [laughs].

GC: Have you any fears?

J: Yes, I have. I would hate to think that I was going to have it on my brain, so that I would have epileptic fits and not know anybody. I would hate that. I hope that I would be able to cope with being doubly incontinent but I don't know if I would. I might have to turn my face to the wall on that occasion.

As Jane deteriorated physically she lost control of her bladder and had to use a urinary catheter, a difficult development for her to cope with. In the second extract below, Jane was at home, confined to her bed and appeared tired of waiting for death to occur. Her conversation was less filled with humour than earlier ones. Her desire for a quick death, however, remained unchanged. Her protracted dying had become an inconvenience and Jane was beginning to think of euthanasia, which she thought would be a welcome relief. Her fears had also shifted; they were centred less on the physical aspects of her condition and more on the metaphysical aspects of whether death was a final process or not.

Case 3 (Jane)

J: I hope it's going to be fairly quick. I don't want to drag it. You can't tell what's going to happen to you. You could be paralysed, you could be ga-ga, really. I could be having fits. You have to take it as it comes, there is nothing you can do about it really.

GC: The last time we talked, you talked a bit about euthanasia. Do those thoughts still go through your mind?

J: Oh yes, definitely. Especially this week because my son is going to Hong Kong for a month with his wife, and my daughter is going to Sri Lanka for two weeks. So knowing my luck, I'm just as likely to pop off when they're out there, which means it will ruin both their holidays.

GC: Jane, in your own mind how long do you think you've got?

J: Not very long, I don't think. Maybe a couple of weeks. I was only given six months and that was two years ago.

GC: Do you feel ready for it?

J: Yes.

GC: Not afraid?

J: No. Well I suppose everybody is a bit. You don't know where the hell you are going.

GC: Where would you like to go?

J: I don't mind where I go. I don't think you go anywhere really.

GC: Do you think it's pretty final?

J: Oh yes. It's got to be, hasn't it? My God, we'd never be able to have all the millions of people who have died.

GC: How would you sum up this experience, Jane?

J: One I could do without. I never knew it was as frightening as I thought it was going to be. My mother has always said that God only gives you pain that you could bear and though I never believed it, I think she's right in a lot of ways. The actual thought of dying is far worse than the actual going. It's so final, though in actual fact I have come to the conclusion that it's not that final.

Jane died two weeks after this conversation as she predicted. She died quietly in her bed, without signs of physical struggle, although her dying was protracted and not a quick death as she wished for. She saw her son before he went to Hong Kong and knew that her daughter had landed that day from Sri Lanka. She also spoke to her mother the morning before she died.

Just as the experience of death of family members is likely to have a profound effect on the attitude of patients who are dying themselves, so too the death of fellow patients may have considerable impact. For instance, Susan (case 1) and Carol (case 2), both knew Jane (case 3) and watched her progressive deterioration and the protracted process of her dying. The marked effect of these observations is illustrated by the following conversation with Carol, who was the last to die of the three patients.

Case 2 (Carol)

GC: Carol, as you know, Jane's died, and Susan too. The three of you were together for some time. How do you feel?

C: The only thing I can think is, I remember how Jane was feeling and the only thing I can feel is kind of relief really for her because she was suffering. I know she said to me she wouldn't mind if she died. I know the feeling if you're not getting any better. But Susan of course was a lot younger but very sad for her. But we've all got to go sometime.

GC: Does that make you look at yourself when it happens?

C: Yes. I often wonder how I'll go.

GC: How do you think you'll go?

C: I don't know. I just hope I'll go in my sleep and I don't know about it.

GC: When these thoughts go through your mind, like they do with some of us, how does that make you feel when you're thinking about death and dying?

C: I guess I'm pretty fatalistic. It doesn't worry me. It doesn't really bother me. In fact, I think: what use am I as I am? I think there must be something better up there than it is here.

GC: Do you believe in that?

C: Yes, I do.

GC: Do you have a religion?

C: Yes, I'm Roman Catholic. I don't really believe in hell or anything. I think you get that here.

Previous exposure to the dying experiences of family members was also important in shaping individual constructions of the manner and mode of death preferences. For instance, Carol (case 2) nursed both her husband and mother when they were dying and used their deaths to construct a model death for herself.

Case 2 (Carol)

GC: How did they die?

C: My husband went into a coma, and my mother had a heart attack and died in her sleep, which was a nice way to go. That's how I'd like to go.

Carol drifted into unconsciousness and died shortly after sustaining a fracture of the odontoid peg from a fall, following a long period of slow physical decline.

As with Carol, Susan (case 1) also wanted to die during sleep like her mother, but not at home. For years after her mother's death she associated her home as the place of her mother's death. Susan did not want her children to similarly associate their house with death. She hoped that, when her time came, it would be a peaceful death. Below is an extract of the conversation we had about her thoughts and desires about death and dying. I asked Susan whether she had given any thought to how she might want her death to be.

Case 1 (Susan)

S: Well, I thought I might be able to come into the hospice. I don't want to die at home, because I can remember when my mother died. She died at home, which was lovely. She died at night in her sleep but I wasn't there, I was away. But every time I went back to the house I felt a bit strange. I don't want my children to feel the way I did.

GC: When your time comes, do you want it to be like your mother's?

S: Yes, definitely. And I feel if I came here it would be like that. Mind you, everybody that's died here has been very old. A man died in the night and he was 87. You can't really be too upset at that age. But they've all seemed so peaceful, so yes, that's what I would like.

Unlike the 'old' patients she mentioned, Susan, who was in her early 40s, died struggling. She was frightened and continued to hold on, despite a rapidly deteriorating body. She appeared unable to leave her young family. She was finally able to let go only after asking her family for their permission to die. Her husband spoke of waiting for her to die, like 'waiting for the birth of their children'. According to him, it was a 'laboured process'. Her death and struggles until the end made a profound impact on the nurses and her family.

These three cases highlight how people draw on previous and current exposures to dying in shaping their desires and preferences for their own. Both Susan and Carol were able to link their construction of a model death directly to personal experiences. However, for other patients who had not been exposed to death the construction of dying and death were based on watching the dying of fellow patients. Looking at death, as in seeing and touching the dead body of a fellow patient, is more unusual. However, this experience may be a positive one, if sensitively conducted, as in Lyn's case (case 5).

The first extract below was from a conversation conducted with Lyn at the time when she started to deteriorate. Lyn described herself as not religious and often talked openly about her thoughts on death. This was mostly based on her experience of watching others in the hospice, as Lyn had no experience of deaths in her own family. I asked about her thoughts of how she might like her death to be.

Case 5 (Lyn)

L: I have never really thought much about it. I just hope that I would just... really I'd just like to go. Like most people would really. I think it takes about a fortnight when it gets really bad, that is what I have worked out through watching other people.

GC: From watching people here?

L: Yes. Seeing people die. You can tell when they are in their last fortnight. You can actually tell when people are in their last fortnight.

GC: How has it been for you, making friends here and finding that some of them do die? How does that affect you?

L: It doesn't affect me too badly, actually, because once people get so ill I think it is nice that they go. I don't get upset by it. It's just the fact that I don't like people kept going in a lot of pain. I think it's nice they go.

The next extract was taken a few weeks before Lyn died. During this time Lyn was able to watch for herself, at close quarters, the period immediately before and after the death of a fellow patient. This experience was significant as it provided her, for the first time, with a model death.

GC: How do you see the future for you at the moment?

L: Not very rosy. I can't think of another way of putting it.

GC: In what way do you mean?

L: It's making it feel like it's more final for me, where everything is going.

GC: What makes you say that, Lyn?

L: I think, because of how ill I've been and I've seen death more in a way. Have I told you about Maureen [another patient]?

GC: No, can you tell me about that?

L: Well, one day I got asked if I could change over my room again, like I quite often do when people are really ill. I changed it over and I didn't know who it was for, but I knew Maureen was in the ward, so I asked if I could see her and they [nurses] said they would arrange for me to see her. It was night time. It wasn't until the next day that they arranged for me to see her. In between time I had gone to her room, seen her door open. I didn't have to disturb her, I just looked through the door and saw Maureen the way she normally sleeps, with her mouth open, peaceful at rest. Then the next day they came to my room and said that they had heard that I wanted to see Maureen but they didn't realise that I didn't know she'd died. So they were ever so tactful, they said that I could still see Maureen if I wanted to but they had a few other things to tidy up before they take me to see her. I said I've never seen a dead body before, so they took me to her and it was lovely to see her at peace. I'd actually seen her at peace in her sleep and she'd died in her sleep. She died so peaceful and she looked so peaceful. It was quite nice in a way.

GC: That experience — did it help you make some sense of it? Is that how you would like it to be for yourself?

L: Yes, I would, but I'm frightened of it being too sudden in case it upsets my son too much or upsets other people. I am more frightened of it upsetting other people than what I am myself.

GC: Lyn, Maureen's example — what did you make from that?

L: Well, that death isn't frightening. She died so peaceful in her sleep and never came around and it wasn't at all frightening. It is very hard to put into words but I got a lot of comfort from it and I'm really glad I peeped into her room the night before. Whether it was right or wrong I don't know, but I don't think they would have minded.

GC: Right now, as you are going through all these thoughts in your mind, what are your feelings? Are you afraid, are you ambivalent or can you talk a bit about how you are feeling?

L: I am not afraid. I've never been afraid so far. The only thing I am afraid of is in case I try to hang on too long, which I think you can do. I am worried in case I drag my life out too long because I don't think it would be any good for me or anybody else — that does worry me a bit, in case I try to drag my life on.

Lyn was in her 40s and, like Susan (case 5), died struggling. She was unable to let go, although her body was rapidly deteriorating. Unlike Susan, who sought and was given permission by her family to die, this did not occur with Lyn, and the pulls of her family for her to keep going became a tremendous strain towards the end. At the moment of her death, one of Lyn's sons threw himself at her, shook and thumped her on the arm and leg, calling for her to return to life.

Although the above accounts show how people appear to shape and construct thoughts about model deaths, they also show that deaths does not always occur according to our wishes. This may be attributed to the multiple facets of dying, which include physical aspects of the disease process, the personal make-up of the individual and his/her relationships with others, which all contribute to shaping and determining the manner, style and approach of the individual's dying and death.

As death became imminent, the emotional intensity of nurses appeared to increase. Often feelings of sadness and wishes for a speedy death were expressed by nurses. These were mostly made with reference to the time and manner of dying. For instance, some nurses made remarks such as: 'I hope she/he doesn't drag on' or 'I hope it's going to be quick, for their sake, or 'She/he wouldn't like it to go on and on'.

The wish by some nurses for a speedy death for the patient appeared to arise from a desire for them and their relatives to be spared the pain of having to watch, wait and experience the anguish of prolonged dying.

Case 6 (Kathy: Alison's nurse)

K: I think, over the last few weeks in particular, seeing her deteriorate and not being able to communicate and her quality of life was very difficult for Alison. She found that very frustrating, being unable to sort of talk to us properly and at times because she was so sleepy as well. I know it's hard to make assumptions about what Alison would have liked but, knowing Alison, I think she wouldn't have wanted to continue much longer like that. So I was relieved in a way that things have happened quite quickly for her, because I don't think Alison would have wanted to linger on and on and on the way things were going. Again that was very hard for her mother, sort of seeing her like that.

GC: What about you, Kathy? Is it difficult for you to watch patients linger on like that sometimes?

K: Yes, it's difficult. I think it's more difficult when you are aware of what the family are going through. I was very aware that it was very hard for her mother. It is a bit of both, on the one hand she doesn't want her daughter to die and wants her daughter, but on the other hand she doesn't want to see her continuing like this. So no, I'm not saying that it sounds like I'm wanting things to happen because it was hard for me seeing her like that, which it isn't at all. I think you are just aware of what the family are going through. I think because you can pace yourself and when somebody actually continues, still hanging on for a lot longer than expected, it gets much more difficult for the relatives to therefore pace themselves. They get physically and emotionally exhausted when it goes on day after day after day, because they don't know when the end is going to come and they are just having to hang on in there. They have mixed feelings they don't want it to happen but on the other hand they are not sure how much they can take. It was getting very hard for her mum seeing her like that.

SHIFTS IN THE EMPHASIS OF NURSING ACTIONS DURING THE TERMINAL PERIOD

As death became inevitable, there were indications that nurses shifted from a supportive role (enabling and supporting the independence of the patient), to a combined 'doing for' and supportive role for the patient. 'Doing for' includes performing bodily care for the patient, including washing, bathing, feeding, assisting with defaecation/micturition and moving the patient. These aspects of care were documented by the nurses in their daily nursing notes and generally increased as the patient's physical condition deteriorated.

Together with providing support for the family, other important desires expressed by the patient, such as the wish to see a relative or friend, or to spend a short period at home with the family, also assumed a greater significance. Respecting the person's needs to tie up loose ends or settle unfinished business was perceived as an important part of nursing care as death approached. Considerable efforts were made by staff and relatives to try to make this possible for the patient. This combined doing for and supportive role is illustrated by James.

For James (case 11), his Christian faith was important to him. During his admission, he was often tearful and admitted that he was terrified of dying. His anguish and distress were also linked to religious questions of whether his life had been good enough and whether there is an after-life. This was related to issues from James's childhood and his past relationship with his brother. These issues had not been expressed before, but as James deteriorated they began to emerge. The following extract showed the effort and role played by James's nurse to help him resolve some of these issues.

Case II (Kevin: James's nurse)

GC: Can you tell me how James is feeling?

K: He seemed to be expressing a whole mixture of thoughts and anxieties related to dying, such as whether he had already died. He would tend to nod off to sleep and then wake up and ask if he was dead. He didn't necessarily recognise me throughout the evening but within about 48 hours he came to call me by name when I approached him. That was partly due to familiarity and partly due to a slight decrease in his confusion, and certainly his confusional muddlement, whatever you like, seems to vary so that sometimes he's pretty lucid. I think it is very important to listen to him carefully because at times I have noticed what seems like being muddled, [is] a kind of expressive dysphasia in that if you unravel carefully what he is saying then it makes sense. He'll think of a word he wants to use but use several words to describe because he can't remember the actual word he wants. I think interestingly, underlying all of this, has been, to me, is his personality. It is quite striking I think.

GC: You mention that in his more lucid moments or not so lucid moments he was talking about whether he was dead or dying or whether he had come back from death itself. Did he talk quite openly about that to you at any time?

K: Not what I would describe as openly. I would say that there was quite a lot of intuition on my part and therefore my interpretation of things is obviously open to question and might even have been completely wrong, but he seemed at various points to be, to have a sort of, I don't know if its quite the right word but existential spiritual distress at things that he'd done in the past and had guilt about. These things were talked about on the surface but there was obviously a great deal more underneath them. There were things to do with his childhood and his brother that may have been causing him distress and Joan [his wife] arranged for his brother Peter to come in and we shut the door and let them spend time alone together. And that seemed to have some therapeutic effect in that following that he did continue for about another day to talk about Peter but then it sort of dwindled and he seemed much more at peace.

GC: Did you initiate this? Did you suggest Peter should come in or was it done by his wife?

K: It was done by his wife, but I think I spoke to Joan a number of times at some length about these aspects of his care because it also involved the visit of a priest, which had to be done carefully because of the danger of James thinking that the visit of a priest meant that we all thought that he was about to die. So I spent quite a lot of time with Joan talking about these issues and whether or not, as it were, putting things in order was a good thing and how one should go about it. I remember a few days after his admission I was in the room with Joan and James and he was agitated about some small thing, I don't remember what, and Joan said to him: 'You've sorted things out with Peter, you've sorted out things in the past, all you need to do now is to exist for the pleasure of your family.' I thought that was a very lovely thing to be able to say to anybody and I think it also reflected on what I was talking about earlier of his personality. I think he was a very strong person, someone who was, is, a very good father, a very good grandfather — he obviously takes great delight in his grandchildren. Another picture I had in my mind is yesterday he had a nine or 10-month-old grandchild in his arms in the bed. I had to go into the room for something but it felt like an intrusion and part of me wanted to withdraw. I needed to check something with Joan and went in. The family didn't seem to feel that it was an intrusion in the same way that I did. I somehow wanted that bond to last as long as possible.

Together with his wife, James's nurses were able to help him settle some of the important issues of his life which he felt were still unfinished. As well as the visit from his brother, James's priest came and anointed him with oil, which seemed to bring some him calm. James died the following week in the presence of his wife. At the time of his death, his eyes were described by his nurse as half-open and he appeared to be in slight distress. His death aroused some misgivings in Joan. She felt that there was still some unfinished emotional business between them, because it was only in the latter days of their marriage that they had begun to communicate on an emotional level. As a result, Joan expressed regret that she had not done this sooner.

'Doing for' was undertaken by the nurses as the patient progressively became weaker, more bed-bound and less alert. These acts were only undertaken when it became clear that the patient could no longer maintain his own physical care or when he specifically requested help. In other words, the patient's independence was encouraged and respected by the nurses as long as possible. This seemed consistent with Lawler's (1991, p.180) contention that the dying were treated differently from recovering patients. For instance, dying patients are allowed by nurses to 'determine more of their level of dependence' (and consequently independence), and generally 'encouraged by nurses to retain as much control as possible for as long as possible'. On the other hand, recovering patients were not discouraged from being dependent. According to Lawler (1991), this dependency, albeit nurse-controlled, was tolerated, along with the view that the sick person usually gets better and returns to social responsibilities.

Depending on the nature of nurse-patient rapport, the performance of physical care appeared to affect the nurse's construction of situations to a greater or lesser extent. For instance, James' (case 11) nurse commented:

Case 11 (Kevin: James's nurse)

K: I've enjoyed the… I suppose it's the rapport, but it's not the sort of witty rapport like you have with some people but James, for whatever reason, is pleased to see me, so I suppose there is… the psychological term is 'stroke'. I may have been 'stroked'. He's quite heavy physically. It's just sometimes when he needs to be transferred out or whatever I feel a sort of weakness come over me.

GC: You mean physically you feel you're not strong enough to lift him? Is that what you're trying to say?

K: The sense of weakness I feel when it comes to moving him from, say, his bed to the commode is just the same as I would feel with any physically heavy patient. I was talking to him earlier about his bowels and I was offering him suppositories because I was told that he had abdominal discomfort and it was particularly bad overnight. So a positive part of me took over in the sense of thinking 'well, if I've got to roll him over and give him suppositories, then get him out quickly onto a commode, then that's good if he feels better at the end of it'. But it's just the physical task that I could happily avoid if there were any other way of doing it.

Conversely in Carol's case (case 2) where the patient was less communicative, physical tasks and 'doing for' were seen rather differently. Performing physical care was seen as a means of getting some response from a non-communicative patient. It fulfilled the need for gaining some job satisfaction.

Case 2 (Val: Carol's nurse)

V: At the end of the day I actually find it easier once I am actually having to physically care for them [patients]. When people actually become really sick and can't look after themselves anymore then the feedback I get is by doing things for them, they respond, even when they are properly sedated. I can still put in physically and you can talk to people even if they are asleep. I think this is probably what I will get from Carol even if she never says anything to me.

From a social-psychological perspective, the interplay between acts of holding on and letting go continued to play an influential part in terms of family and personal attachments during the terminal period. Nonetheless, the pace of bodily deterioration remained a key element as regards whether the person could continue to hold out against death. For some, these attachments and 'holds', set against a rapidly deteriorating body, appeared to contribute to a situation of 'not knowing how to die'.

PATTERNS AND MODES OF DYING

Close analysis of the cases during the terminal period revealed that, contrary to claims in the literature (see Chapter 2), both patients and nurses consistently separated body from personal self, and the nurses used this construction as a way of assessing the trajectory of a patient towards death. These findings are illustrated below by reference to selected extracts from interviews with the nurses.

Patients' and nurses' constructions of body-person split and readiness to die

In most cases, as a patient's physical condition deteriorated, he/she attempted to separate the body from the personal self, and a similar phenomenon was observed with the nurses. This was demonstrated by the language used by both groups in redefining critical situations and changes. In the case of patients, the body-person split was observed to occur when they talked about their physical condition or preparations for their funerals. The first extract from my conversation with Peter (case 12) shows how he defined his situation in order to cope with dying.

Case 12 (Peter)

P: Somehow I find that I think I have got the right attitude for me to cope with this illness. It doesn't worry me and I can accept it, but perhaps that is because somehow my body seems to enjoy illness. I don't, so this is just one of the things that I have got. If I catch something else, it won't particularly worry me.

Peter also talked about how he would like to dispose of his body

P: I will donate my body to help other people. What about the main frame of my body? If people want to take something from my body then as far as I am concerned they can take the lot. By the time you've taken the kidney, the liver, you can go on and on, but if it is used to help somebody else, then that's what I would like.

In contrast, Ian (case 4) expressed his desire for a cremation.

Case 4 (Ian)

GC: Ian, we were just talking about whether one should have a cremation or a burial. What are your thoughts on this?

I: My personal thoughts would be that I would rather be cremated, because in many ways it's better, it's cleaner and it takes up less space for the body. Whereas if you are buried it takes up a lot of ground waiting for someone else to die to come and join you there. I think it is much better to be cremated.

While patients' separation of the personal self from the body seemed to occur when talking about their disease, symptoms, or as part of funeral arrangements, in contrast, nurses' construction of the body-person split seemed linked to gauging whether the person's physical and personal self were in synchrony when confronting imminent death. Various references were made as to whether the person or their body were ready to die, as illustrated by the extracts below.

Case 12 (Ruth: Peter's nurse)

GC: You mentioned so long a wait. What happened there?

R: He just plateaued out and was waiting for weeks and weeks. He was ready but his body had then recovered and so he wasn't ill enough.

Case 12 (Sally: Peter's nurse)

GC: So Sally, in terms of looking after Peter and his dying, what do you make of it?

S: As he wished, which was living life to the full if you can call it that, right up to the last day and he was one of these people who sort of used the expression 'dying on their feet' except he was on his bed, but he really didn't give in until his body just refused to carry him any further, I think.

Case 5 (Lesley: Lyn's nurse)

GC: So, Lesley, thinking of Lyn's dying, did you feel she was ready for it?

L: I think at that point she was ready. I think in the weeks leading up to that her body was physically very, very weak, but I think, mentally, spiritually she wasn't ready to let go. The only way I could describe the weeks leading up to it was like a wounded animal who was just desperately trying to get up all the time and just couldn't rest and couldn't be at peace. She was just fighting, fighting, but I think that morning we actually reached a point where she actually made it very clear she'd had enough. She was ready to let go, she realised she was dying. She just wanted to be out of it, she wanted to be less aware. So I think we reached a point where mentally and spiritually she was ready to let go but unfortunately the family were not at the same point.

Similarly, Alan's (case 10) nurse made the following observation on gauging whether Alan's personal and physical selves were both ready to die.

Case 10 (Miriam: Alan's nurse)

GC: Did you feel he was ready to die?

M: I did feel he was ready to die, yes. He said to himself: 'What I have got to live for?'. As far as he was concerned he enjoyed coming here to see everybody and see his friends but there was nothing for him at home. He used to really dread going back home to an empty house. He was a very private man and when his wife was alive they were a very private couple, they kept themselves to themselves. They didn't have many friends and when she died a large part of life had gone and he said that there was nothing that could replace that. He was offered bereavement support but he said: 'What can they do?' rather than 'okay, I can talk about how I am feeling and how much I am missing her but nobody can actually replace her'. My feeling was that yes, he was ready to die. He had no fear about dying, that's the time when he would be with his wife and that's what he wanted.

When asked whether she thought Alan's physical condition matched his personal desire to die, Miriam replied: 'Physically no. When I heard that he had died I was actually quite surprised. Certainly over Christmas I hadn't sort of thought: oh, Alan's going to die very very soon, because physically he had deteriorated each admission but I didn't feel he was going to die yet. So that did come as quite a surprise.

This separation of the physical and personal selves in gauging the synchrony of dying appeared to be used by nurses as a way of redefining and conceptualising whether the patient was ready to die. It appeared to serve several functions. Pragmatically, it provided the means for nurses to pace their preparation for the patient's death, thus being better able to meet the needs of both the patient and their relatives. Conceptually, it provided a mechanism for unravelling and understanding the emotional and physical complexities of the phenomenon of dying. Therefore, the construction of the body-person split appeared to provide the nurses with a 'practice-orientated conceptual map' for understanding the patients' readiness to die at a critical juncture of the dying trajectory.

Nurses' conceptual map — four modes of dying

The nurses' construction of the patient's state of readiness to die can be represented by the following four patterns:

- person ready, body not ready;
- person ready, body ready;
- person not ready, body ready;
- person not ready, body not ready (Fig 9).

These patterns are defined by the shape, duration, expressions and manner of dying. Any patient could exist in one pattern at a time but could change between patterns, depending particularly on their physical condition but also on their acceptance of the imminence of death. The ways in which the patients either remained within one of the four patterns/modes of dying, or changed between patterns, is highlighted on the opposite page.

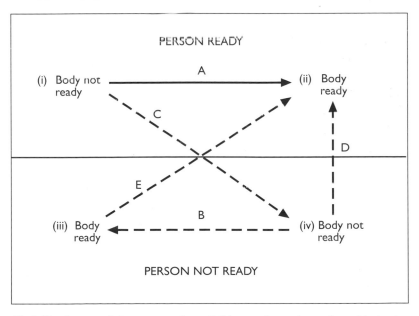

Fig 9 "Readiness to die" – conceptual map. Solid arrow shows observed transition, and dashed arrows show potential transitions

▨ Person ready, body not ready

This pattern of dying applied to cases 2, 3, 6, 10 and 12. The patients appeared mentally prepared to die and, as in the case of Carol (case 2), Jane (case 3), Alan (case 10) and Peter (case 12), said overtly that they were ready to die. However, their bodies did not comply, causing the death to appear slow and prolonged. This is illustrated by the conversations I had with the patients' nurses.

Case 2 (Val: Carol's nurse)

GC: Do you think she is dying now?

V: Not immediately, no.

GC: How do you see it, your gut feeling?

V: She has said herself that the APD [pamidronate treatment] is no longer effective. She has spoken to her friend and said she has had enough and she really can't fight this anymore and I think that physically, and in some ways she is relatively strong. I don't think she has really got the mental energy any more to keep going much longer. But I think she is keeping going more for her son than anything else really.

Case 3 (Karen: Jane's nurse)

GC: Do you think Jane's dying was in keeping with her desire of the death she wanted for herself?

K: Well, Jane implied that she wanted to die sooner, really, rather than later. I was there at the end of last week and she was weaker but not dramatically different. When I was sitting with her she was obviously breathless but not distressed by it and I said to Ron a couple of times when I was leaving, 'I think she's quite poorly', and he said: 'I see a change each day.' She had been ready to die for a long time.

Case 10 (David: Alan's nurse)

GC: David, what was Alan like during the last few days here?

D: Looking after him wasn't that difficult really. He seemed to go down very very quickly and I think an element of it was surprise.

GC: His surprise or yours?

D: He was surprised; but I think his surprise was moderated by his lack of will to live. He had some episodes where he wasn't feeling so good but these seemed to pass; they weren't followed by any other symptoms. He seemed to be a wee bit concerned about them, he didn't want to go home and tackle them there. But once things seemed to move on, they seemed to manifest in other ways and his breathing picked up and there was more weakness, he seemed to accept things. He actually said to one of the staff at one point: 'Just let me die.' We have been obviously his contact with the ward over the last few months. He is obviously a lonely person, very very cut up about his wife's death, and I think he just reached a point where I imagine some other people would have thought: hang on, what's going on? This is an acute condition that I have got. Alan almost seem to say: 'Well, fair enough, if it's an acute condition then it doesn't really matter, it will happen fast.'

It is important to note, however, that while accepting that their deaths were imminent and inevitable, patients such as Alison and Peter (cases 6 and 12) continued to resist the finite nature of their situation by using denial-like mechanisms. Nonetheless, as their physical condition deteriorated, both these patients lapsed into semiconsciousness and died quietly without struggle.

Of the next extracts, the first shows Alison's grief and her expression of not being ready to die (although she was fully aware of her impending death), and the impact this had on the nurse caring for her. The second illustrates the nurse's account of the events surrounding Alison's death.

Case 6 (Debbie: Alison's nurse)

GC: Does she ever talk to you about her dying at all? Does she see her deterioration as part of her dying?

D: Yes, she does. She doesn't talk about it too openly because Alison never has. She is still very, very frightened and angry about what is happening. There is a tremendous amount of anger inside Alison at the moment because she does see it, but her way of actually acknowledging to me was the fact that she had had this dream of her father and he was calling her and she said: 'I'm not ready yet, Debbie, I don't want to go.' I said: 'I understand that, Alison, I know how you feel.' We are doing everything possible to get her back on to a better plane but things have gone wrong and she did acknowledge this. We did talk fairly deeply about it, that things were going down and things weren't so good and she did then want to block it after that conversation. She had lost her mobility, she had lost every chance that she thought of independence, and I think that one of her biggest fears was the fact that she was frightened that she wasn't going to go home.

GC: Clearly there are times when it must be hard work for you. How do you cope with that?

D: Oh yes, it is because she also throws everything at me because I am in that role of a nurse and I find it very hard. I come out of a session with Alison sometimes feeling totally shattered and want to cry my eyes out. But she always makes up for it, because she always afterwards says sorry. She knows what she has done, that she has really hurt me. She knows that she can use me, but she does, and it takes a bit out of you, but she always afterwards, always, without any doubt, grabs my hand and says 'sorry', or just gives me a squeeze and I know that means sorry. It helps tremendously.

Similarly, Peter (case 12) appeared to cope with his dying by using denial-like mechanisms on a daily basis. The following account highlights how Peter's nurse ascribed meaning to the manner of Peter's approach to his death.

Case 12 (Ruth: Peter's nurse)

GC: Ruth, there was a period of time when Peter sat up and said that he was waiting to die. Have you got any thoughts about that?

R: I think Peter had reached the stage where he was ill for so long and he had pretended to himself that he was going to get better and then he sort of decided that he had had enough of pretending and he wanted to be real, and he said: 'I am going to die.' And he knew he was going to die and he wanted it because he had gone through the process and reached the conclusion that he wanted it to happen, and he wasn't really ready for it to be so long a wait. It was nice to see the positive aspect in that he was able to talk to Joyce and tell her things that he had wanted and hadn't been able to, like how he wanted his funeral and what he wanted her to do, and that was very positive and very good because they had never been able to do that before. What was sad was that he just didn't die and I think he really believed that once he decided he was ready to die he would die and then he didn't, and he didn't cope with that at all well.

GC: How do you respond to that when you see patients and the processes of dying operating in front of your eyes? How do you care for these patients?

R: You just have to give them time to talk about things that are worrying them because some days he would want to talk about why he wasn't dying and other days he wouldn't. You just had to be there and not misinform him or mislead him and just be honest and say: 'Well, it does take time' and not say: 'Well, yes, you should be dead.' It will be when it's ready and not when you are ready.

Person ready, body ready

This pattern may be applied to the same patients listed above (cases 2, 3, 6, 10 and 12) and denotes a phase entered by them when their physical condition began to match their personal readiness to die.

The nurses' accounts below illustrate the events prior to the patients' deaths.

Case 2 (Pam: Carol's nurse)

GC: Can you describe what happened to Carol?

P: She was very withdrawn After she had sorted out her funeral plans with Mike, her son, she appeared more at ease. She wanted to go gently and she achieved this. She was ready for it and her body had kept on going for so long. There was no struggle, and that was nice for her. Val and I laid her out. Her face looked terrible, not like her glamorous self, but after we washed her and dressed her in her pyjamas she looked more at peace and that was nice for her son, who was very affected by it all.

GC: Do you think that's how she wanted to die?

P: Yes, I do. She was very much on her own really. The only man she loved had died and she came back here to be with her son whom she left years ago, so it was right for her when the time came.

Case 3 (Karen: Jane's nurse)

GC: How would you describe her death?

K: Very peaceful. No change in medication. I'd spoken to Dr Smith on Thursday, saying what if she is more poorly and not able to swallow her co-proxamol because she was finding it difficult? He suggested we might use some Benoryl, and Mandy, who was on at the weekend, knew what our thoughts were. But I was a bit concerned that because there were so many drugs that she couldn't tolerate that the end might be quite difficult. In particular she'd been breathless, chesty and had pain problems at times and a lot of problems with her catheter. I did wonder if the last phase of her illness would be particularly difficult, but it obviously wasn't. Ron was relieved in many ways that it had been so peaceful, although obviously devastated, and he says there is so much missing because so much of his life in the last several months has been involved looking after Jane.

Case 10 (David: Alan's nurse)

GC: When did Alan die?

D: He died on Thursday, at 9 o'clock. It seemed to be very very easy, it wasn't a struggle at all. To begin with he seemed, as the changes were happening, he was obviously anxious about what was happening to him. But a lot of the times, although he was breathing very fast, he didn't say he was breathless. He said he felt weak but he just rested on the bed and in the event it just seemed like he just made some sort of decision to say: 'Well, what will be will be' and there was no evidence of resistance or animosity, anger — any sort of negative emotions. It was very sort of accepting and 'go with it'.

GC: Did you think he was ready to die?

D: Yes, I think Alan was probably ready to die a long time before he did. Having watched him from outside and seeing Alan prowling around his room and the look on his face. His life had ended with the death of his wife and there was no way he was ever going to get anything back. For him to be with her was his wish. Obviously taking his own life wasn't an option.

Although Alison (case 6) and Peter (case 12) resisted the inevitable nature of their situation, as their physical condition deteriorated both of them were observed to lapse into semiconsciousness and died quietly without struggle.

Case 6 (Lesley: Alison's nurse)

GC: Lesley, I'd like to ask you what happened — if you could describe the events leading up to Alison's death and what sense you made of it?

L: I was on duty over the weekend as Alison deteriorated. On the Saturday morning she was much more sleepy and didn't really wake up until lunch time. When she came to at lunch time she actually had a good afternoon. She was actually quite alert, she had lots of visitors with her and even though she couldn't communicate verbally she was actually able to communicate very well otherwise. Her facial expressions made it very clear what she wanted and what she didn't want. She had a good afternoon, enjoyed having her family and friends around. It was almost like she had her last fling really. As I went off duty on Saturday afternoon I was aware she was also getting a little bit chesty. Apparently that got worse over the evening and overnight. When I came back on the Sunday morning she was actually very, very chesty but she was now unconscious. Alison deteriorated very quickly during that morning, didn't respond at all, didn't really come round at all and deteriorated very quickly and died in the early afternoon. Her mother was with her, and I and a close friend of hers and her brother who had arrived a quarter of an hour before. Her mother felt it was actually quite a significant thing. Her father had died three years ago and it was actually his birthday that day. So her mother felt it was quite significant that day and felt she was going to die that day and that was right.

Case 12 (Sally: Peter's nurse)

GC: Can you describe what happened when Peter died?

S: Right, well, in fact the night staff reported at 7.30 this morning that he had had quite a poor night and several times they thought he was actually dying and as we were having the report one of the night nurses came into the office and said that in fact they thought we should call the family because he had deteriorated further, which we immediately did. We went in to see Peter, that is myself and a bank nurse, two bank nurses actually, and you could see that Peter really hadn't got very long to live. One of the night nurses, Cindy, stayed with him for about five minutes and then we took over. He was very, very peaceful.

GC: When you say peaceful, what do you mean?

S: He was calm and was, I suppose, semiconscious, lying quite still and breathing shallowly and not distressed in any way.

GC: Was he able to acknowledge anyone or was he unable to?

S: No, he wasn't, he was virtually unconscious by this time and very much towards the end of his life. We stayed with him and one of the nurses remained a further 20 minutes, and by 8.30 he had died peacefully without regaining consciousness. His wife arrived shortly afterwards — about 10 minutes — with Peter's daughter, and they have been here all morning, getting support and encouragement from various members of staff.

▦ Person not ready, body ready

This pattern was quite different from the previous two and was characterised by patients who appeared to hold on to life despite bodies that were in rapid physical decline. Dying appeared to be a struggle for all four patients' and their deaths were often described as 'difficult'. This way of dying applied to cases 1, 5, 9 and 11.

Despite their unreadiness to die, when it became clear to them that, physically, they could no longer go on, two of the patients (cases 1 and 5) eventually asked for sedation to help them cope. The accounts below described the patients' manner of dying and events leading to their deaths.

Case 1 (Jean: Susan's nurse)

GC: Jean, tell me what happened.

J: When she came in on the Friday she seemed fairly well in herself. She was still mobile and still up and about. She came in with the hopes that she would be having a blood transfusion and that would have some miraculous effect, even though she knew that the last time she had one that hadn't happened. It took quite a while to actually get her blood transfusion. The blood was lost, it went to the orthopaedic hospital and that was really upsetting for her. She had to wait about 24 hours before she got the transfusion. She had the blood transfusion and it didn't seem to make any difference at all. That almost seemed to be the point where she started to go down.

GC: On the Friday?

J: No, on the Saturday. She had the blood and things didn't seem to be working. Then the doctors decided perhaps an epidural infusion would help the pain. She went over to the oncology ward to have it. As she arrived, Dr Smith decided that her platelets were too low and went over herself to tell this to her. Then Susan came back and was very agitated, seemed to want to sleep and was asked: 'Do you want to sleep?' She said: 'Yes, I want to be more sleepy'. So early in the afternoon she had a dose of midazolam.

GC: Did she ask for that?

J: Yes. She had a dose of midazolam, went to sleep, woke up about two hours later, talked for a while then said to me: 'What I want is to be asleep, as I was with the midazolam'. So we said that was fine if that's what she wanted. So we gave her another dose of midazolam and she very quickly — well, it wasn't so much a sleep — but she was extremely relaxed and that's what she wanted. She was still aware of what was going on because she could respond to questions. Apparently that afternoon her husband and daughter came in and Susan asked permission then from both of them if it was alright for her to let go now.

GC: All three of them?

J: No, she asked James and then she asked James to ask the children if that was okay. I think he just asked Jane because she was there and they said yes. They gave her the permission. I wasn't there again until the Monday morning. I came in on the Monday morning and she was unconscious, breathing very rapidly and had a nasty faecal discharge from her mouth.

GC: Was she aware of it?

J: I don't think so, no. We moved her into a side room with the explanation that it was nicer, not only for the family to have that privacy but also for the other patients, because she was making a lot of respiratory noise.

GC: Was she very noisy?

J: Yes. And that was quite distressing for the relatives as well as for the other patients. We moved her in the middle of the morning. James stayed with her, Tony the eldest son was there, Jane was there, the youngest son was not there. He had come in on the Saturday to see her and literally ran out and decided he didn't want to come back. He actually went out with his friends the day his mother died. She was breathing extremely rapidly and was given IV diamorphine to try and control her, but it didn't work for very long. She seemed to be in pain from what we could tell. We just kept increasing her midazolam and her diamorphine accordingly.

GC: How did she die and what happened to the family?

J: She died about lunch time from what I could remember. James called me just literally seconds before she died. We were having to suck her out quite a bit. She was actually bleeding as well as having faecal fluid coming out of her mouth. We gave her some nasal suction. I was particularly worried that she was going to vomit and die, haematemesis or whatever. James called me in, I asked him to excuse us for just a minute, I was in there with the doctor and while he was out of the room she died. So we called them back in immediately and said to them that she's died. He was very concerned for the children.

GC: How did that leave you feeling?

J: I found it very distressing. I was quite distressed by it because partly of her being young, partly because I didn't have a very good relationship with James and none of us on the ward did because he had been very self-contained, and therefore we didn't feel we were supporting him very well. I found the daughter the hardest.

GC: Why was that?

J: Because she was saying like, a quarter of an hour after her mother died: 'I'm going to drive home now' and I was saying: 'You're not in a fit state to drive home' and she was saying: 'I'm perfectly alright'. Yet you could see she wasn't at all and her father was saying: 'Look, I'll come home with you,' and she's saying: 'No, I'm alright.' She was in a numb state and couldn't get through to her at all, and I was very worried that she was going to have an accident. When James left he went to find the youngest son who was somewhere down town with his friends.

GC: Would you say Susan died the way she would have wanted?

J: No.

GC: How do you think she would have wanted it?

J: She would have hated to be leaking faeces out of her mouth. She wanted to go to sleep and she wanted to die in that way. I think she would have liked it to be a bit quicker, which is what she had expressed before. That would have been less distressing for her family because especially James was really distressed by the leakage from her mouth and the dyspnoea.

Case 5 (Lesley: Lyn's nurse)

GC: Lesley, do you remember that particular morning when you saw Lyn? She was very ill at that time and you talked to her about how you were going to plan her care? Can you tell me a little bit about that?

L: Just to give you a little bit of a background to that morning: Lyn had an absolutely dreadful night. She had a horrific nightmare, very vivid, which was absolutely terrifying for her. She had been so terrified she had actually been sort of scared to close her eyes, because every time she did she started this nightmare. She was absolutely terrified and by the morning she was absolutely exhausted and when I came on duty she was sort of sitting on the chair in the centre of the ward where we usually sit. She was exhausted, she could hardly keep her eyes open, but still clearly very, very scared. This nightmare — I don't know if you want to know about the nightmare — but she was still, you know, having vivid memories of the nightmare and was actually sitting there thinking that she was actually covered in blood, which was sort of quite terrifying. Anyway later we sort of helped her back to her room — she wanted to go back to her room and then Lyn actually made it very clear that she was actually quite exhausted. When I was discussing with her how she wanted us to be able to sort of help her and what she wanted to do she actually made it very clear that she'd had enough. She said: 'I can't go on any longer like this. I've had enough and I just want to sleep and I just want to have a long, long sleep and not the sort of sleep where I have been sort of drifting off and waking up. I just want to have a long, deep sleep.'

So then I discussed with her how we could actually help her to sleep and discussed with her that we could actually give her something that would help her sleep and have a deep sleep. I discussed this on previous occasions with Lyn and she had always made it very clear that no, she didn't, she wanted to be awake, she wanted to be in control, she didn't want actually to have anything to help her. But at this point she made it clear that she'd had enough. She'd had enough of living and just wanted to be less aware, so that's where we came to an agreement. We gave her some midazolam to help her settle, but that involved negotiating again with the family too, because they were very much wanting her to be awake until the last minute.

Dr Smith and I both felt that perhaps we had to relax more, once she was actually more sedated, but nature may take its course and she may actually then deteriorate quite quickly. We felt the family ought to know, although what we were doing wasn't in any way hastening her death, but it may in a way just be giving death a chance. Again that had to be negotiated very carefully because the family weren't ready for that and they were wanting Lyn to go on for as long as possible and they were wanting her to be alert and awake for as long as possible.

GC: What was the response when you saw them?

L: It was a mixed response. Lyn's younger son was there and his response was actually nothing at all. He couldn't respond, he didn't know what to say. He was just full of tears and he actually couldn't speak, it was very very difficult for him. I actually spent quite a bit of time… I allowed him time to sit on his own and just to think about things first of all and then I went back to see him. Both Dr Smith and I had both seen him together to explain the situation. We then left him on his own for a while and then I sort of went back to him and spent quite a bit of time with him. And again he found it very difficult to actually say what he wanted and how he perceived things. I found the only way I could really communicate with him was that I actually ended up saying: 'Is this how it seems? Is this how you are feeling?' and he would either sort of say 'yes' or 'no' and that was the only way I could actually get any indication of how he was feeling. After some time he did make it clear that he did understand that his mother was dying and that, yes, although it was very difficult, he didn't want her to die. On the other hand he wanted his mum to have what she wanted and he wanted her to have peace and some rest.

GC: What about the other son?

L: The other son at this time actually wasn't around because he hadn't actually been involved up until this point. Lyn's partner had been around and I discussed all the same things with him. Again it had to be negotiated very carefully — what we were doing. I also rang up Lyn's parents and asked them to come in so that we could speak to them. It was actually quite easy with Lyn's parents because they actually wanted, I think they were finding it all too difficult and, unlike the son and partner, actually wanted to see Lyn more at peace.

GC: This was all done before the drug was given?

L: Yes, which again was quite difficult because of time. But we felt we couldn't do anything until we actually got their blessing in a way because we felt we had to work together with them. It was eventually agreed that we should do that and Lyn had some midazolam and she settled down quite quickly and then she slept, not as long as we thought, but she had about four hours' solid sleep. It was nice because she then woke up quite refreshed and feeling much better in herself. She'd had no vivid dreams and she woke up feeling quite different about things. She was awake for a short time and then asked again, she wanted to settle down and wanted to go back to sleep again and then she had some more sedation and actually then slept right throughout the night.

In contrast, the situation for the other two patients in this group (cases 9 and 11) was less clear cut. This may be attributed to a number of factors. For instance, Ted (case 9) was admitted to the local acute hospital as an emergency 'terminal admission' and therefore was not in the hospice. He was not openly vocal and was reported to have considerable pain. He appeared to be alert and fighting until the end. James (case 11) was muddled and unable to communicate. He seemed restless, agitated and in anguish, and sedation was given.

Case 9 (Diane: Ted's nurse)

GC: Diane, you mentioned you'd like to read some notes from your reflective diary about Ted's death?

D: I actually found looking after Ted extremely stressful and distressing. I have never come across someone alive or dying where the pain has been so difficult to get under control. It's awful that it took six days to get his pain under reasonable control. I wish I had been more assertive with the doctors and got them to listen to me. Philip, one of the doctors, was good, and I suppose it was my lack of experience as a nurse which did not help. I suppose, because I had no definite idea where Ted's pain was coming from, that was more difficult to actually establish what we should actually use. What I found most upsetting was when we were turning him, because he just froze and I thought he was going to start screaming out. We found it very difficult to turn him, even when we got three or four of us — he was still in so much pain, he really was. I was glad that he died when he did. His necrotic scrotum was swollen and looked so painful. I thought of giving him more analgesia than I should do — it did cross my mind because he looked so in pain. His scrotum had gotten more black as the days had gone on and the tumour had started to come out of his rectum as well. The whole thing, you watch somebody go through this... I felt extremely guilty that we didn't turn him on one shift. I suppose it was the thought of inflicting him with so much pain when we turned him, and then thinking it out, I thought we should have turned him because had he developed pressure sores it would have given him more pain. I felt his pain was under better control, but I didn't know whether it was because he was more comatose than anything else. We had music and aromatherapy going on in his room and he had his own pyjamas on. He was freshened up and given clean sheets. We were able to tidy him up and make him look more comfortable and feel more comfortable. The only thing I do regret about the day he died was that there was nobody in the room with him when he died. It was very unfortunate — it was just one of those things when we had actually gone out of the room just to change his syringe. We didn't actually get any warning because he didn't actually Cheyne-Stoke or anything like that. He just went very quietly and very quickly. I didn't actually feel that upset. I was glad in a way that he was out of pain, that he wasn't suffering any more. I didn't actually feel like crying. I find I get very close to my patients and I normally do cry with the relatives or when they do die. I suppose I didn't feel that close, I only looked after him for about six days. Perhaps because I didn't know the real him, I didn't get close to his family either, something else which normally upsets me when somebody dies, probably because much of my contact was over the phone or just a few brief words, because they didn't stay that long. I could understand in a way why they didn't stay. I don't think I would like to remember somebody who looked like that, with that smell. Perhaps I didn't build up close ties, although I felt my care was good.

GC: Can you sum up what sort of death Ted had?

D: I think he died in a way that he shouldn't have done. I think he should have been more peaceful and I don't know whether the smell bothered him at all. He didn't actually say anything at all, even when he was awake. That could have been something that could have worried him and I felt that we should have done something about that earlier. I think we should have had his pain under more control before he died. I don't know whether he felt alone because there was nobody there with him when he died but he was quite comatose. He wasn't Cheyne-Stoking, he was still breathing very strongly. He wasn't chesty or anything like that. He didn't get bubbly as they can do. I don't think he was very aware of what was going on nearer the end.

Case 11 (Kevin: James's nurse)

GC: Can you tell me what happened?

K: I believe it was diamorphine and midazolam, and the diamorphine was given because he had chest pain, and the midazolam because he was extremely agitated and restless. Again, looking at the history of events which in a sense I can look at objectively, because I wasn't here for the time that all this happened. I gave him the last lot of tablets that he took Sunday lunch-time and went off duty. I was off Monday, Tuesday and came back Wednesday, yesterday, when he died. Joan had been home for Sunday afternoon and this injection had to be given while she wasn't here. The nurses who were here held back waiting for as long as possible for Joan to return, because they were well aware of the need to consult with her. In the end, for James's comfort they had to go ahead and give the injection. I think she felt a great sense of guilt having not been here at a particular point when he, as she saw it, needed her. She felt had she been here she could maybe have prevented this injection being given. She maybe could have calmed him. The previous day he had some chest pain which had settled with Asilone and she felt perhaps if she had been here she might have been able to sway events so that he could perhaps have lived for another day or two, remain conscious for another day or two. This is leading into a third area of concern — that there was still unfinished emotional business between them. It was only in the latter days of their marriage that, as Joan put it, they started to communicate on an emotional level and, as I said, there were still things that were on her mind and she wanted to deal with. One of the things I suggested to Joan was that, although James was unable to speak to her, there might be things that she could say to him, and I think over the next few hours that she did speak. She said she had already been doing that and I think perhaps she did that a little more in the few hours before he died.

GC: Were you present at the time of death?

K: Yes, throughout the afternoon James's breathing was quite strong and although he was peripherally shut down and it was clear that he hadn't got very long to live I thought during the evening that he was going to live into the next day. So I decided on that basis that I should turn him because he had been lying on the same side for a few hours and I wanted to make sure that his skin condition and so on was okay. After turning, he deteriorated very rapidly and died in about half an hour. I stayed with Joan throughout this time. If I hadn't had the good strong basic relationship that had already formed between us, I'm not sure what I would have done at that point, but it felt right. Although she said nothing to me, her concentration was very much on James. She held his hand and there was an intensity in the way that she looked at him and studied him. Somehow there was almost a link through the air. I can't quite describe it. Something based on the intimacy of years and years of knowing somebody. At the point where it clearly was going to be only one or two minutes before James died, I discreetly left because I felt that they needed that particular moment alone. I think Joan perhaps wanted to tell James that she loved him, perhaps one or two other things as well. She wasn't a person I felt who needed a third person as a supportive presence at that point. She was, in a sense, strong enough and experienced enough to be there alone.

■ Person not ready, body not ready

In contrast to the above patterns of dying, three of the patients (cases 4, 7 and 8) continued to hold on in a physically stable condition while their disease remained in remission. As this happened, they began expressing more confidence in planning their future.

Case 4 (Laura: Ian's nurse)

GC: I think you've got some concerns about how Ian is being treated, like he's been in and there's talk about trying to get him into the disabled unit. Do you want to comment on that?

L: Yes, I've been thinking about Ian and I have felt that I have encouraged Ian to be too accepting with his situation because it has been a very difficult situation for him. He's had so many different things he's had to cope with besides his cancer. Now that the cancer he's here for is in remission, and people are saying perhaps he's cured from this, we're now thinking that he should be more rehabilitated and concentrate on doing more for himself and perhaps thinking that the pain he is suffering all the time really is his main problem now.

Case 7: (Laura: Margaret's nurse)

GC: Can you tell me how Margaret is and how you find caring for her?

L: Margaret is really well at the moment. She's feeling quite energetic, sleeping well, eating well, and she's managing to get around and getting her confidence, although she always takes a stick with her when she goes to town. She goes out for coffee regularly now and I think it's wonderful. There's a remarkable change in her.

GC: Just think back what was it like before, compared to now in your care for her?

L: Well, she was quite demanding. She always liked to be, when she was very ill at one stage and needed a lot of care, but now I really don't need to spend an awful long time with her because she just says how well she is all the time. There's a great difference.

GC: In herself, do you notice a difference as a person?

L: Yes, I think there is. She says she doesn't try to hurry herself at all. She just takes life as it comes and she takes about a quarter of an hour getting dressed. She says that's fine, she's not in any hurry.

Case 8 (Laura: Sheila's nurse)

GC: Laura, can you tell me what has happened to Sheila since we last met?

L: I think at the moment she is really wanting to stay at home more. She has had a very bad chest infection and this has made her feel very weak, and she just feels she needs time at home. She has only been coming to the day centre once a week.

GC: She seems to be someone who is very afraid when she sees people dying around her. Can you tell me a bit about that?

L: When she came in last week she was really absolutely devastated to hear about Louise and then afterwards to be told of another patient who had died. She was in tears and she really felt terribly upset about it and she said: 'I really quite dread to come in to be told this'. I discussed this with her and I said: 'You would prefer that we did tell you about it, wouldn't you?' and she said: 'Oh yes, of course, but it is just that I never know who is going to have gone next' and that is absolutely devastating for her. She was very, very upset last week.

GC: How do you think she copes with that?

L: I think at home she goes over it quite a lot. I think also it reminds her perhaps of her father's death whom she was very fond of — she actually had to come from Australia to just be there in time. She also said that she really misses him terribly because he was somebody who, well, her mother was apparently 'up and down' quite a lot, rather like her perhaps, but he was very steady and she relied on him.

These three cases exemplify a situation where the patients' physical condition had stabilised and, despite being initially prepared for a poor diagnosis, their confidence grew with time. They were engaged in surviving and not in dying. This gradual change in their condition raised questions about the nature and location of their care. This included the need for the patients and their nurses to redefine the role of the patients and to re-accommodate this change in enabling the patients to cope with long term survival.

Summary

In this chapter some key patterns and styles of dying have been defined. In particular, a person's state of 'readiness to die' appears to involve an interplay between the acts of 'holding on' and 'letting go'. The mismatch between bodily deterioration and the patient's desire to hold on generates anguish, conflicts, tensions and sorrow for the patient, family and nurses. Important influences on this interplay include family attachments, the extent of physical incapacity and the psychological accommodation to withdrawal from the present life. Religious beliefs did not appear to be any more significant than the other factors in determining the pattern of the terminal phase of life. In studying the cases it became evident that the days leading to death are fraught with complexities both from a treatment/care perspective as well as from that of family relationships. Even when it is possible to manage symptoms physically, and to enable the dying person to be less anxious through the use of drugs, relationship issues may be difficult or impossible for the people concerned to resolve. This may contribute to much anguish and spiritual unease for the dying person and members of their family.

The notion of a peaceful death is commonly used by staff to describe the ideal and, indeed, is the death desired by most people. Nevertheless, despite the best possible medical and nursing management, a peaceful death may remain impossible for some patients. As the case studies show, some deaths occur without much struggle, whereas others occur with considerable struggle. The term 'peaceful death' implies that the individual is at peace with the situation from physical and psychosocial perspectives. It is debatable whether the expectation of a peaceful death can ever be realistically achieved for many people, given the complexity of the psychosocial issues present, as demonstrated in these case studies.

The very variable state of a person's readiness to die has been described in detail. In studying the cases it was clear that, as the disease progresses, distinctions are made by both patients and nurses in separating the physical and the personal aspects of the patient's make-up. This separation of body from personal self, or body-person split, appears to be significant for nurses in constructing an understanding of a person's style, pace and mode of dying. The pace of bodily deterioration remains a key element regarding whether the person can continue to hold out against death. Four patterns of dying have been proposed: person ready, body not ready; person ready, body ready; person not ready, body ready, and; person not ready, body not ready. For some of the patients, a mismatch between their attachments and 'holds', on the one hand, and their rapidly deteriorating body on the other, contributes to a situation of not knowing how to die. However, for the three surviving patients, how to adjust to living is clearly an important one and posed new challenges related to management and care. Within this context of death and dying, tensions, anxieties and conflicts appeared to co-exist with satisfaction, joy and reward in the experiences of both patients and nurses.

III: Dying and nursing

9. Conclusion: implications for nursing practice, theory development and future research

REDEFINITION OF SELF
AND THE PROCESS OF DYING

Using Denzin's (1992b) interpretive interactionist framework, I have taken the stance in this study that experiences of problematic situations rupture routines, disrupt lives and provoke radical redefinitions of the self (Strauss, 1959). Recent studies have shown that problematic situations — for instance, a life-threatening illness (such as diabetes, heart attack or cancer) — is likely to serve as a prompt for continual examination of the self (Charmaz, 1983; Gullickson, 1993; Jones, 1993) and frequently results in redefinition of the self (Lynam, 1990). For instance, Lynam demonstrated that people view cancer in the context of its influence on their abilities to fulfil social roles or in terms of how it changes their social relationships. According to Lynam, this perception is instrumental in terms of how contextual elements and dynamics of relationships are perceived as supportive by cancer patients.

This study showed that individual accounts of dying can be used to provide an important means for understanding the relationship between problematic situations and the redefinition of the self during the experience of dying. In all the cases, constant redefinitions of the self appeared to occur for the patients at each critical juncture of their experience. This phenomenon appeared to influence the way nurses respond in gauging the 'pace' of the patients concerned. By being exposed to the experiences of people facing impending death, nurses in the study were involved directly and indirectly in the plights of the people in their care. They made regular references to their attempts to gain insight and understanding into the feelings and actions of the patients at critical junctures. The nurses often repeated key phrases used by patients to describe their situations, as well as adopting the stance of viewing critical situations from the 'eyes of the patients'.

Thus, nurses in the study used patients' constructions and redefinitions of selves as cues in determining the patients' pace and meaning of losses (or gains) incurred. This formed the basis for decisions on actions of nursing care to explore with the patients concerned. The meanings constructed from problematic situations at each critical juncture provided the basis for the continual redefinition of the self, by the individuals concerned and, at the same time, the patient-nurse/nurse-patient relationships appeared to be constantly defined and redefined.

There has been little research on problematic situations and their potential to provoke radical redefinition of the self, in nursing studies of death and dying. Therefore, considerable scope exists for future studies to develop and clarify further the relationship between dying patients' construction of the self at critical junctures and nursing responses in delivering care. This approach also has important implications for nursing practice and education. It directly challenges the non-critical application of procedural nursing frameworks (such as the nursing process) that attempt to objectify, predict and control nursing problems. The process of dying in this context is far more complex than is implied in nursing process frameworks. It requires the direct involvement of individuals, the recognition that individuals engage in the process of redefining at critical junctures of their illness, and the ability of nurses to take part and engage in their patients' redefinition of selves.

PATIENT-NURSE/NURSE-PATIENT RELATIONSHIPS IN THE CONTEXT OF DYING AND DEATH

A key methodological interest of this research was to gather data from practice to provide a prospective account of both patients' and nurses' construction and management of their experiences in confronting impending death and the trajectory of certain death, but at an unknown time. The study showed that within the context of providing and receiving care, complex, subtle strategies and interplays were used by patients and nurses in pursuing and maintaining relationships. It has also shown that such relationships are dynamic in nature for both the patient and nurse and, moreover, a considerable amount of knowledge can be obtained from studying situations in nursing practice. As highlighted in the preface, although nurses are well placed in matters of dying and death, studies of patient-nurse encounters and the constructions and actions that arise out of them are seldom pursued in nursing studies.

In this study, patients and their nurses continually appeared to engage in a process of 'encountering'. This can take a multitude of forms, such as direct face-to-face contacts (in attempts to construct and elicit meanings of particular situations), or direct and indirect actions of planning, or manoeuvring situations behind the scenes.

Conflicts, tensions and rewards between patient, nurse and families were endemic. The acts of protecting and controlling, watching and waiting, holding on and letting go provided some key dialectical elements in furthering the understanding of complex strategies and interplays acted out in order to cope with continuing losses. This study provides a broad basis for an understanding of the interactive processes and interplays between patients and nurses. Clearly, further prospective studies of a similar kind are required to explore, refine and test specific themes and concepts raised here.

Nurses in the study appeared to provide both empowerment, guidance and respect for patients without negating the self-worth of the people concerned. Nursing practice, in this sense, often involves taking risks within a fine balancing act which comprises pacing care, doing for or covering up to prevent embarrassment. The nursing emphasis on encouraging patient control and independence is a significant one and appears to be related to expectations of outcomes. Faced with the prospect of death as an outcome for the dying person, and 'dependence' as the dying person becomes more incapacitated, it was not surprising that a sense of urgency and the need to maintain the dying person in an independent and normal state for as long as possible were evoked in most of the situations described in this study.

However, an important finding relates to the ability of some of the nurses in negotiating a plan of care with the patient about their dying when death was clearly imminent, by providing choice (such as whether to remain aware or sedated), at the same time as respecting the patient's wishes and remaining with them regardless of their decision. This ability exemplified skilled expert nursing care and has implications for the individual concerned in determining their own way of dying, family members and their perception of the death of the patient, and nurses and staff, in whether the death of the individual was well managed. This particular aspect of death management will clearly benefit from further studies on decision-making processes at this crucial time of the patient's dying and the notion of how nurses and staff encourage individualised death in institutions.

The study also provides further support for the view that 'care work' (James, 1986) is both emotionally and physically labour-intensive. The continual encountering between patients and nurses has a deepening effect on their relationship. The nursing act at the time of death is a symbolic one: nurses are seen as taking part in enabling an individual to make the transition from the present world to another (however that other world may be construed). When a patient's death was imminent, grief and sadness were often expressed by members of their families, nurses and other patients. Difficult deaths, such as when patients struggled to hold on to the attachments of the present life, make the dying process of some people painful and difficult for the nurses and families to watch. This particular phenomenon is seldom made explicit in nursing discourse and theories. It clearly has implications for how nurses manage the emotional aspects of their work and how health care organisations support staff who are exposed to these experiences. In particular, it raises the issue of 'closure' as part of the process in concluding care for dying patients (Smith, 1992). Further research is required to clarify the concept of closure, to identify specific acts of closure and to examine the ways in which nurses and patients use closure in their relationships.

At a practice level, this study supports the view that patient-nurse encounters appear to be conducted within the context of individuals' personal construction, actions and meanings of personal situations in confronting death and dying.

While recent attempts have been made to identify the types and nature of nurse-patient relationships in nursing, generally the focus of such work has been solely from nurses' perspectives. In the messy world of nursing practice a perspective comprising solely of nurses' views is clearly limited. Providing nursing care involves patients and nurses in a relationship that is 'layered' and 'sequential-relational', so nursing practice is seldom clear-cut. It requires a detailed understanding of the process of dying, the culture in which dying is located and the ability of nurses to balance providing care with the emotional aspects of the work.

PHYSICAL, PSYCHOLOGICAL AND SOCIAL INFLUENCES OF DEATH AND DYING

One of the main areas of focus in this study was to describe the multi-dimensional aspects of dying, taking into account the influences of physical, psychological and social interplays, including the individual's family life-cycle. Importance was placed on the background and identity of the person and on their physical, psychological and social situation during the process of dying. As discussed in Chapter 1, the prospect of facing impending death inadvertently engages them in watching the impact of this physical process on their own body. This clearly affects their social relationships with others.

Physical

The nature and extent of body deterioration are crucial in determining the individual's quality and length of life. As I followed the patients there was evidence of a range of physical incapacitation, such as weight loss (or gain, from the use of steroids), fatigue and weakness, breathlessness, incontinence, loss of speech and pain. Although some of these symptoms may be managed and reduced, for most of the patients it was only a question of time before the body became overwhelmed by the disease process. Watching the body physically deteriorating and having to cope with an altered body and its products, such as odour, sputum, leakage of fluids or faeces, vomit and bleeding was unpleasant for everyone concerned. Fortunately, for most patients, the moments of death were often preceded by lapsing, or being enabled to lapse, into a state of semi- or non-awareness. This bodily deterioration leading to death is well captured by Nuland (1994, p.142), who stated that 'by and large, dying is a messy business'.

The impact of bodily deterioration therefore affects not only the person concerned but those around them. Moreover, each new pain, weight loss or symptom was carefully watched for and, by some, construed as significant in terms of the disease progression (even though this may not have been the case). The nature and extent of bodily deterioration (or lack of further deterioration), constitute an important influence on the construction and manner of dying or surviving. The latter, as indicated by three long-term survivors in the case studies, has posed new challenges in caring for long term cancer survivors. For two of these patients (cases 4 and 7), their continued survival with advanced cancer has created tensions in terms of the continued use of an expensive service and the appropriateness of the place of care. Similar tensions may well have arisen with regard to the patient in case 8, had she not voluntarily decided to reduce her contacts with the hospice for other reasons. For the staff concerned, a conflict arises between wishing to use expensive resources most effectively and not finally discharging patients who are in apparent long-term remission, in case there is a relapse.

The required psychological adjustment to survival has been topical in recent years, following reports of experiences of cancer survivors (Tross and Holland, 1989). The emotional leap from the status of dying patient to survivor clearly raises implications for hospice nursing, where the goal of care — preparation for death — is diametrically opposite to one of survival. This finding has implications for the ways such patients are supported and enabled to make the transition to a survivor role. It poses challenges for both the nurses faced with direct care-giving and the organisation that has to provide resources for the care-giving. For instance, organisationally, policies for discharging cancer survivors and long-term support are still largely undeveloped. More importantly, the needs of such patients and the ways in which they can be helped to make the transition from a dying to a non-dying role require urgent study.

Psychological

The findings of the study appeared to support the recent contention that psychological factors, such as denial and acceptance of dying, fluctuate in varying degrees throughout someone's dying trajectory. Denial and acceptance appeared to be used as strategies to avoid threats as well as to preserve existing relationships. In contrast to some commonly held beliefs, which tend to view denial and acceptance as singular, either/or entities, this study highlights the need to view denial and acceptance as interdependent strategies, used continually by patients. Indeed, use of these mechanisms did not conform to set mechanistic stages as indicated by Kübler-Ross (1969) in her stage theory of dying.

Moreover, denial and acceptance are important psychological mechanisms. They were used during the process of reframing and constructing meanings at critical junctures and through that, for the radical redefinition of self, in coping with a problematic situation. On occasion, the meanings which the person constructed for themselves could be acceptable to them but at odds with those of the people around them. This was particularly so when a person's construction of their situation did not match their physical condition. In this situation, instead of preserving relationships tensions often arose, as seen in Peter's case when he talked about his role in future events when his death was clearly imminent. Weisman (1972) refers to this denial as 'third-order denial': people have accepted the facts of their illness and are facing imminent death but occasionally resist the finite nature of their situation. Clearly, this has implications for the ways nurses manage such situations in practice. For instance, while realising that there are dangers in colluding with the patient, there is also equally the need to recognise that the patient who is aware of his dying needs the occasional indulgence in not having to confront his mortality. It is important, therefore, for educational programmes on communication with dying people to consider situations where they may use denial as an appropriate strategy to cope.

The nurses in the study appeared to engage in a series of fine balancing acts in their encounters with the patients and their relatives. In particular, tensions occurred when patients exercised control by not talking openly about their situations or by talking in ways that were inconsistent with their rapidly deteriorating condition. It was clear that, for some, there was a need to engage in different levels of awareness. This appeared to relate to how people confront their mortality, psychologically, on a daily basis. Thus it has implications for practice. Although nurses may work in settings where a culture of open awareness prevails, this may be deceptive with individual patients. For example, some patients may use coping strategies, including denial, which may not fit with health care workers' ideals and expectations of open awareness.

Social

Contemporary literature has highlighted the social processes that characterise the trend towards death and dying in institutions, including hospices. Although my study was located in a hospice, the social world of the individuals was by no means confined solely there. The hospice served as a focal point for encounters between patients, their families and professionals. For most patients, the hospice provided an added dimension to the patients' social world: at one level, this was concerned with matters related with living and, at another, the concerns were issues of dying and death.

There were no indications that Sudnow's (1967) concept of 'social death' featured in the social context of the hospice. This was unsurprising, as the hospice philosophy and culture centre on enabling people to engage in life and living. Interestingly, Mulkay's and Ernst's (1991) portrayal of how some people may be perceived as 'socially dead' by some parties but 'socially alive' by others appeared relevant, albeit paradoxically. For instance, some attributes of social death occurred through the individual choice of the patient (cases 2, 3 and 11) rather than an assignment of those attributes by others. As physical deterioration occurred, Jane (case 3) and Ted (case 9) chose to remain at home rather than travel to the hospice day centre. This choice limited their social contacts to family and close friends. Moreover, Jane's loss of mobility meant that she was mainly confined to her own room in her home. Her social withdrawal became more pronounced as she became weaker, when she began to wish that her visitors would leave. Similarly, Carol (case 2) chose to remain alone for long periods in her home and when admitted to the hospice she often chose not to engage in the social activities offered. This was due partly to increasing weakness and the desire to preserve energy for her son's visit These patients' choice to withdraw socially from the world of hospice life, and life in general, appeared to create conflict for some of their nurses. This may be related to coping with perceived rejection by their patients, holding the view that 'dying people are to be encouraged to engage in living while dying' as opposed to disengaging from life, and being genuinely concerned for the patient.

While many patients used the facilities offered by the hospice, not all expressed a desire to die there. For those who wished to die at home, the expressed desires were sometimes unfulfilled, particularly where either their physical condition or family circumstances, or both, made it impossible. Three of the 12 patients were explicit in their wishes to remain at home. Of these three, one (case 9) died in an acute hospital ward following emergency admission, and another (case 8) voluntarily reduced her contact with the hospice and continued living within the notion of surviving. Only one patient (case 3) was able to fulfil her wish of dying at home. In this particular case considerable efforts were made by the hospice and primary health care teams to achieve this by providing comprehensive home care support.

At the face-to-face level, the notion of 'collective' dying in such a hospice was clearly an issue for some patients. Watching dying and deaths (both as a spectator and as someone experiencing the process itself), appeared to evoke fears, distress, sadness and feelings of guilt, as succinctly described in the accounts of some patients. The tension between being a spectator and as someone experiencing the dying process was managed in several ways. Some chose not to get involved with other patients, some reduced contact with the hospice and others overtly expressed feeling upset.

For other patients, however, being able to observe the care provided to those whose deaths were imminent appeared to provide some reassurance (Honeybun, Johnston and Tookman 1992). And, as exemplified by case 5 (Lyn, who had never seen a dead body before), the sensitivity shown by the nurse in allowing Lyn to see the body of a fellow patient who had died and looked at peace clearly helped Lyn construct a less fearful picture of death. According to Lyn, she gained a lot of comfort from the experience. It is doubtful, however, whether a similar outcome would have occurred had a less peaceful death scenario been presented — such as in case 1, whose death was not only difficult but also 'ugly' (with faecal discharge). Paradoxically, Lyn's dying was a difficult struggle, extending to the moment of her death, with her son violently thumping on her chest in his attempt to revive her.

The actions of nurses and other health care professionals are clearly important in influencing patients' constructions about the process of dying. The demonstration of 'attentive caring' further reinforces the view of that care should be based on belief in the self-worth of individuals, despite a deteriorating and diseased body. The extension of this care until and after the time of death provides reassurance for those patients who are present during the dying process but who have not been exposed to previous deaths. There has been little previous research on the impact of death on fellow hospice patients. Further work in this area may yield important data on the concept of 'collective dying', which will have considerable implications for nursing practice and future research.

While death and dying are unique individual experiences, they are also interactional and dynamic. Each person's experience can influence others' construction of living with impending death and the process of dying. These face-to-face experiences can also extend beyond the presence of patients and staff to wider society, via the families of patients. Family members may also have to redefine the self in coping with a problematic situation such as the death of a loved one, in order to reorganise and redefine relationships within the family. The encounters between professionals, patients and their families are thus potentially crucial processes, particularly in contributing to the transitional phases of family life cycles.

Overall, the social organisation of dying in the study reflects the culture of this particular hospice setting: it operates on both institutional and personal levels. It is a unique blend of what I call 'personal-institutionalised care', clearly deviating from the impersonal, inhumane experience of dying observed in some institutions. Arguably, when seen at its best, it exemplifies humane institutionalised care for the dying that incorporates many advantages of the family-centred death at home, but with expert nursing, medical and other professional care on hand.

IMPACT OF DYING ON THE PERSON

It became evident that philosophical aspects of existential 'loss of self' was an important concern expressed by the patients. Sadness and grief were often expressed in response to the losses accompanying disease progression and physical deterioration. Often the expressions of grief were related to previous, current and anticipated losses. The study provides some preliminary qualitative findings to support Aldrich's (1963) postulation that not only the bereaved but also the dying experience anticipatory grief.

Although the dying person's grief is commonly seen, research on the grief of dying people is limited, compared to research on the bereaved. In particular, the concept of 'anticipatory grief' (Parkes and Weiss, 1983; Rando, 1988) and its impact on the dying person remains largely unexplored in nursing. Much has been written about concepts of loss and grief (for reviews, see Littlewood, 1992; Stroebe, Stroebe and Hansson, 1993; Copp, 1996). However, the term 'anticipatory grief' has been criticised as a misnomer (Rando, 1988) because it suggests grieving for anticipated losses, rather than for past and current losses which, Rando asserts, are often the source of the grief. In defending this argument, Rando (1988, p.71) states: 'In contrast to the implications inherent in the term "anticipatory", which suggest that it is solely a future loss that is being grieved, there are, in fact, three time foci toward which anticipatory grief directs itself: past, present and future. In the experience of grief undertaken between the receipt of knowledge of fatal diagnosis and the actual death, that period traditionally seen as encompassing the time of anticipatory grief, the grief that is experienced is actually stimulated by losses that have already occurred in the past and those that are currently occurring, as well as those that are yet to come.'

My study provides evidence of the existence and experience of anticipatory grief in practice and lends support to Rando's (1988) argument that viewing anticipatory grief as a unitary concept is an oversimplification. In reality, anticipatory grief is multidimensional, spanning two perspectives (patient and family), three time foci (past, present and future) and three influencing variables (psychological, social and physiological). Clearly there is a need for future work to explore the phenomenon from the perspective of the person who is dying, develop and clarify the concept of anticipatory grief to include the dying, and examine the relationships between past, current and future losses as constructed by dying people.

MANNER OF DYING

By including personal identities, and individuals' connections with past, present and future events, the study has been able to capture the multifaceted nature of the manner of dying. Specifically, the influence of time and the progression of disease appeared important in terms of how patients constructed their thoughts and wishes about the manner of their dying and death. It appears that the manner of a person's dying and death is shaped by the approach taken by them and this determines the style of their death. In all 12 cases the manner of dying was unique for that patient. This was particularly so in cases 4, 7 and 8 where the patients continued to 'hold out' against death. For instance, the dying trajectories of these patients shifted from certain death but at an uncertain time to one where impending death become less certain. Moreover, thoughts and wishes about preferred deaths were often expressed. These included quick deaths, peaceful deaths and a death that comes without further suffering and incapacitation. These views appeared to reflect the views held by society in general. However, the manner, style and approach of dying (and death) were not always peaceful and were sometimes prolonged, with continued physical deterioration and struggle. Contrary to popular belief, an individual's readiness to die does not appear to be age-dependent — that is, older patients are not more accepting of death than younger people. Rather, a combination of physical, psychological, social and family factors appear to play the most significant role in shaping the manner of a person's dying (Lichter and Hunt, 1990; Lichter, 1991; Twycross and Lichter 1993).

These findings on the manner of dying have direct relevance for nursing practice and education. In my experience, nurses who work in hospices commonly cite 'helping patients to a peaceful death' as one of their motivations. Clearly, the goal of peaceful death is desirable. However, this goal is often unattainable and unrealistic, for those patients who die as well as for those who survive. It is important that nurses caring for the dying are provided with clinical and educational opportunities to explore more critically the concepts of peaceful death and survival.

Theoretically, the study has contributed further towards the concept of a specific dying trajectory — certain death but at an uncertain time — by examining the nature of dying within this trajectory. However, further work is required to understand the manner, approach and style of a person's dying and death in more detail. For instance, it may be useful for future work to incorporate personal identities of individuals and their role within the family life-cycle and focus solely on the influence of these factors on the dying process. Further investigation is also required to examine the trajectory of long term survivors in hospice settings.

PATIENTS' AND NURSES' CONSTRUCTIONS OF 'BODY-PERSON SPLIT' AND 'READINESS TO DIE'

In interviews with patients and their nurses, references were made to the 'body' as separate from the self. Some patients talked about their bodies in relation to disease process and preparation for funerals. Interestingly, as death became imminent, the nurses appeared to 'separate' the person's body from the personal self. The constructions of a body-person split were made by direct reference to the body as a separate entity from the person. As the physical body deteriorated and death approached, this construction gradually became more explicit in the language of the nurses. This phenomenon clearly departs from the notion of viewing the body and self as an integrated being, which has been adopted by nursing in general and by hospice nursing in particular.

The construction of body-person split as death approaches is interesting in view of the considerable amount of philosophical discussion that has emphasised the existential aspects of embodiment. Protagonists of the pro-embodiment view are opposed to the dichotomy between mind and body and argue that the self and body should be seen as a combined whole (Merleau-Ponty, 1962; Shalom, 1989; Csordas, 1994). However, there is also the view that the body is both an object and a subject. For instance, Sartre (1958) perceived the body as 'being for itself' as well as a 'being for others'. Harre (1986) argued that while a person may own a body, he/she also exists within it, so any adequate construction of the body requires an integration of the object-body as thing with the lived-body as experience. Recently, Jackson's (1994) research on patients in a pain unit showed that patients both objectify and subjectify their bodies and pain when using everyday language to describe their experiences. Jackson argued that the legacy of Cartesian dualism of 'matter-over-mind' and 'mind-over-matter' does not adequately describe the lived experiences of patients in constant pain. Patients in her study talked about the pain as an object. The body, another object, had the pain.

Similarly, evidence from Lawler's (1991) study on the management of body by nurses showed that, contrary to currently espoused theory of holistic practice, nurses actually practise in a somological way. Lawler (1991, p.215) coined the term 'somological nursing' to describe 'a style of practice which integrates lived experience with the object body'. Lawler argued that 'somology is not necessarily holistic', although it could be. It is related to the person, context-bound and involving a common-sense definition of holism. According to Lawler, the interaction between the 'body-self dialectic' has long been proposed by Turner (1984) as crucial to our understanding and development of a theory of the body.

During my conversations with the nurses it was quite common to find that some appeared to provide accounts of somological nursing practice being used. These nurses made direct reference to separating the body from the self of individuals. The physical body was then contrasted with the personal self. Whether the two components were in harmony or not determined the patient's state of readiness to die. These findings suggest that nurses use shared meanings to construct an 'everyday working framework' or 'conceptual map' to make sense of the patient's situation when death is imminent. It remains unclear why nurses and patients separate the personal self from the body. It is likely that people construct this separation as part of the process of ensuring a sense of continuity and meaning after death. For although the embodiment of self (personhood) makes a person unique during life, death is finite in terms of bodily human existence. What remains is essentially a body and memories about the individual. An absence of a separation would constitute the total annihilation of the person, body and self.

This particular aspect of the empirical material enables a synthesis of the individual manner of dying to be drawn. This has the potential of being both a useful conceptual map for guiding nurses and for providing a stimulus for future theories. This 'readiness to die' conceptual map (see

Chapter 8, Fig 9) is characterised by the following four patterns of dying: person ready, body not ready; person ready, body ready; person not ready, body ready; person not ready, body not ready. Patients in the first mode (person ready, body not ready) were observed to move into the second mode (person ready, body ready). Although in this study transitions to other modes of dying were not observed, theoretically it is conceivable that such transitions do occur. These potential transitions from one mode of dying to another are illustrated in Figure 9 by arrows b, c, d and e. Indeed, it seems likely that one or more of the three surviving patients (cases 4, 7 and 8) made the transition depicted by arrow c in fig 9, since they changed from a state of readiness to die, having been diagnosed with terminal cancer, to a state of unreadiness to die, having gone into long-term remission. The four modes of dying, combined with the acts of protecting and controlling, watching and waiting, holding on and letting go, while redefining the self at critical junctures, are instrumental in shaping the state of an individual's readiness to die.

The body-person split and readiness to die constructions provide an additional dimension to current theoretical conceptualisations about dying. In particular, they highlight how such real-life situations are managed conceptually in practice. Although current theories on death and dying have focused on elements such as individuals' reactions, awareness, time and duration of dying (Glaser and Strauss 1965; 1968; Kübler-Ross, 1969; Pattison, 1977), the notion of separating body and self as a paradigm for understanding the manner and readiness of dying has not been raised and clearly requires further research.

LIMITATIONS AND CRITICISMS OF THE STUDY

The study is limited in several ways.

Theoretical generalisations

This study was exploratory and aimed at generating theory. It was designed specifically to explore patients' and their nurses' experience of death and dying in a hospice. Patients were diagnosed to have incurable cancer and were aware of the prognosis. The study was therefore biased towards discussing death by cancer in a hospice and did not address dying in other settings or from other incurable illnesses. This clearly limits the theoretical generalisations which can be made.

Depth and scope of study

The use of case studies provided a flexible, open-ended approach to formulate concepts and theories grounded in concrete human experiences. While these have advantages, there were also disadvantages. For example, discipline was required to maintain a balance between the depth and scope of the study. Thus, not all questions raised from the literature review could be pursued. In particular, while psychological influences of denial and acceptance were explored, other psychological responses such as anger, projection, bargaining and hope were not pursued. This has limited the scope of an exhaustive understanding of the influences of other psychological responses during dying.

Similarly, the impact of dying on nurses, although important, was only dealt with from the perspective of 'nurse-patient encounter'. Latent effects of this encountering, and how nurses deal with their emotions following the deaths of patients whom they have cared for, were not pursued. And because the study was designed to gather primary data from patients and their nurses only, the views and experiences of the families were derived from secondary sources and were not the expressed views of the people concerned.

The use of interpretative methods

The use of qualitative approaches in research has been subjected to considerable epistemological and methodological debate (Hammersley and Atkinson, 1983; Lincoln and Guba, 1985; Bryman, 1988). Interpretative methods such as the ones used in this study are therefore not without their problems. Such problems have been discussed at length elsewhere (see, for example, Hammersley, 1992; Miles and Hubermann, 1994). However, it is important to raise the main issues encountered in the study that have particular practical relevance in data collection and analysis.

One of the main criticisms levied against interpretative methods concerns the issue of reliability and, consequently, validity of the data. For instance, in this study data were obtained using interviews and participant observation. Such techniques are open to question and have been discussed extensively in other studies (Melia, 1987; Field, 1987). Face-to-face interviews carry the risk of 'researcher effect' on the interview process and the nature and extent of patient disclosure. In other words, the style and approach of the interviewer may affect the information gathered

(Dijstra, Van Der Veen and Van Der Zouwen, 1985). Moreover, in this study, as a nurse I was already an insider, familiar with the context of the setting and work. The role of participant observer was therefore not difficult and I was privileged to receive a considerable amount of information through natural conversations.

However, inside knowledge carries an additional problem in that I was not a naïve observer. Interpretations of situations may be coloured by my past experience and risk jumping to preconceived conclusions about events or presenting a positive view of nursing actions and motivations. In addition, nurses and patients may wish to present me with a positive view of nursing. Additional steps were therefore taken to counteract the researcher effect by checking information obtained with the participants on a previous occasion each time a follow-up interview was conducted. Additional documentation, the nurses' observations, as well as that of other staff, helped to check the reliability of my own constructions of events as well as those of the nurses.

While these measures helped to overcome some of the potential flaws of interviews and participant observation, the analysis of the interviews, background data and presentation of the findings may also be open to criticism regarding reliability. For instance, it is easy to fall into the trap of presenting the most impressionist phrases from the interviews (May, 1978). A systematic approach was used to code the raw data and care was exercised to provide a balanced account of the findings. Nonetheless, interpretive methods also rely on creativity on the part of the researcher to present new insights and ideas into everyday taken-for-granted human experiences. This is, by nature the *raison-d'être* of qualitative work. Thus, the final interpretation or storyline presented in this thesis will ultimately have to be judged by the extent of its truth value, applicability and consistency as an emergent theory on death and dying.

IV: Appendices

Appendix 1: Focus and design of the study

CONCLUSIONS ON RESEARCH IN DEATH AND DYING: AREAS REQUIRING FURTHER STUDY

Several clinical and theoretical conclusions may be drawn from the reviews on death and dying in Chapters 1-3. Although much progress has been made towards understanding this complex area of human physiology, psychology and social interaction, it is possible to highlight areas of research that are markedly deficient. First, there is a decided lack of empirical studies on the experiences of patients who face impending death, particularly from a nursing perspective. It is often acknowledged that nurses provide continuity of care and thus contribute to the experience of the person who is dying. Furthermore, both patients and nurses possess a wealth of 'practice knowledge' which most are willing to share. However, the nature of the nurse-patient relationship remains largely unexplored. I have attempted to redress this gap in nursing knowledge by conducting an open-ended study in a clinical setting in order to gather information and to capture the dynamic nature of nurse-patient relationships within the context of death and dying.

There is also a lack of studies in which information on physical, psychological and social aspects of death and dying are collated and analysed concurrently. Previous studies have focused either on discrete factors, such as physical symptoms, specific fears about death and dying (and their effects on health care professionals), or social processes of dying and death from organisational or interactional perspectives. A major drawback of this fragmented approach is the general absence of a synthesis of the multidimensional nature of the process of dying. For example, although it is generally acknowledged that physical deterioration occurs when a person is dying, the relationship between physical deterioration and its impact on the psychosocial well-being of the person has yet to be explored. More specifically, how people locate and redefine themselves as they watch the disease progression, and consequently construct meanings about life, remains largely uninvestigated. In reviewing the psychological aspects of dying, it appears that some people use denial-like mechanisms as part of their coping, despite appearing to accept knowledge of their imminent death. This aspect of coping with dying, used in the face of physical deterioration, can be argued as indicative of the process of redefining problems. This act, and its impact on nurses, have yet to be studied in depth. In this study, the influence of the physical, psychological and social aspects on the process of individuals' continual defining and redefining of themselves when faced with impending death are presented.

A third area of deficiency is the dearth of prospective studies. Most of the previous work drew on experiences either of authors or of nurses interviewed by them. I have presented a prospective account and analysis of the experiences of patients and of their nurses. For instance, what were the issues that might concern people who are cared for (or provide care) within these contexts? More specifically, how did they manage their living with the knowledge that they are dying? What were their daily experiences of living and dying? A study of this kind can identify distinct elements and patterns of dying and produce detailed descriptions and analyses of patients' and their nurses' experiences. Further insight and understanding of these issues may provide nurses in practice with a basis for further discourse and for challenging and critically analysing nursing practice in the care of the dying.

Fourth, previous studies do not reflect the open awareness culture of hospices. This is because most of the studies were performed in the 1960s and 1970s when hospice culture was in its early stages and open awareness culture had not developed to its present state. In the literature on the social aspects of dying, the key focus for much of the last three decades has been on issues relating to institutionalised death and dying. Hospice care has, on the whole, been viewed as providing the model of a good institutionalised death, particularly if dying at home is not an option.

However, the ways in which patients and their nurses construct and manage the physical, psychological and social aspects of the dying process within the hospice culture has not been described.

In the past decade, the impact of the hospice movement has greatly influenced the increasing move towards an open awareness culture in health care settings. There is also good reason to believe that this shift in the culture of care has led to an increasing number of people living with the knowledge of 'certain death at an unknown time' (Glaser and Strauss, 1968). The greater openness of staff and willingness to discuss a terminal prognosis means that many more patients are aware of their impending death. Such changes also put the staff member in a different relationship with the dying person and have implications for how someone manages their own dying. This manner of dying in an open awareness culture requires further exploration. Professionals need to view coping with dying as involving not only awareness of events and challenges but also efforts to deal with them, as reflected in the theoretical postulations of Corr (1992).

My research was located in a hospice where patients and nurses interact in an open awareness context and where most patients live in the knowledge of 'certain death but at an unknown time'. The study was influenced by Glaser and Strauss' (1965; 1968) and Strauss and Glaser's (1970) seminal works on the interactive processes and interplays between nurses and patients. However, unlike their studies, my work aimed to explore those interplays directly from the patients' experiences and, indirectly, by the experiences of their nurses. Empirical data from case situations in the study were used to extend and clarify two specific aspects of death and dying theory — Glaser and Strauss' (1965; 1968) 'open awareness context' and 'certain death but at an unknown time'.

Purpose of study and research questions

The purpose of the study was to describe, explore and explain the experiences of patients who face impending death and of the nurses caring for them, in combination with an exposition on current theories of death and dying. To this end, the research questions were purposely broad in order to provide the range and scope for an open-ended inquiry. They were as follows:

- What are the experiences of patients who face impending death and those of the nurses who care for them?

- What is the relationship between the experiences of these patients and the responses of the nurses?

- How are these experiences on dying and death constructed, construed and managed between patients and nurses?

- What theoretical propositions of death and dying are generated from the case situations in practice?

- What is the relationship between propositions generated from case situations in practice and current theories on death and dying?

- How are these propositions different or similar between practice situations and current theories?

In posing the above questions my intention was twofold. First, I wanted to identify key factors and issues faced by patients during the living-dying interval. This would serve as the basis for generating distinct patterns and relationships constructed by patients and nurses. Second, I intended to use the data from the cases to explore and explain theoretical relationships within the 'open awareness' context and 'certain death but at an unknown time' trajectory.

Design principles of the study

As a response to the deficiencies in previously published work, the main design features that were incorporated into the present study are summarised below. This thesis therefore describes a study that is:

empirical — gathering data from a clinical situation;

prospective — following the experiences of a group of patients and their nurses during the living-dying interval;

multidimensional — encompassing the influences of physical, psychological and social interplays;

based in a hospice — exemplifying the open awareness culture of clinical practice and, above all;

viewed from a nursing perspective — including patient-nurse interactions.

Philosophical and theoretical framework of the study

A symbolic-interactionist perspective within an interpretive interactionist framework (Denzin, 1989b; 1992) was used as the philosophical and theoretical framework for the study. Goffman's (1961; 1971) works on face-to-face relationships and the presentation of self provided the theoretical guidance for articulating both the process and dynamics of patient-nurse and nurse-patient encounters as they unfolded. Similarly, Denzin's (1989b; 1992) synthesis of the different forms of self (phenomenological, interactional, linguistic, material, ideological, and as desire) offered a framework for understanding patients' continual defining and redefining of selves in relation to personal identity and relationships with others. This act of redefining problems was seen as central to understanding the way people construct and manage 'critical junctures', an approach that has seldom been adopted in previous studies. Strauss' (1987) and Corbin's (1986) method of coding was used to generate theoretical concepts from the experiences of the participants. This combination of approaches within the interpretive interactionist framework provided the medium for illuminating aspects of personal and structural relationships.

RESEARCH APPROACH USED IN THE STUDY

Rationale for selecting the case-study approach

After careful consideration, the case-study approach was chosen as the one most likely to illuminate how people construct meanings of death and dying from real life experiences. Definitions of the case study vary widely (Lincoln and Guba, 1985; Hakim, 1987; Hammersley, 1992; Ragin and Becker, 1992; Robson, 1993; Miles and Huberman, 1994). Hammersley (1992; p.184) defines the 'case' as 'the phenomenon (located in space and time) about which data are collected and/or analysed and that corresponds to the type of phenomena to which the main claims of a study relate'. Examples of cases range from 'an individual person through a particular event, social situation, organisation or institution, to a national society or international social system' (Robson, 1993). Yin (1989, p.23) defines the case study as 'an empirical inquiry that investigates a contemporary phenomenon within its real-life context; when the boundaries between the phenomenon and context are not clearly evident; and in which multiple sources of evidence are used'.

Traditionally, it has been the view that case studies are appropriate for the exploratory phase of a study; surveys and histories are suitable for the descriptive phase and experiments are needed for explanatory or causal stages (Yin, 1989). However, Yin has pointed out that it is more appropriate to view these different strategies in a pluralistic way, with each strategy being useful for all three stages of a study: exploratory, descriptive and explanatory. Yin stated that experimental work can serve an exploratory function and, conversely, case studies can be both descriptive and explanatory. This led Yin to propose that the best way to choose a research strategy is not to adopt a traditional hierarchical approach, but rather to select a strategy that takes into account the following three conditions:

- the type of research questions posed;
- the extent of control an investigator has over actual behavioural events;
- the degree of focus on contemporary as opposed to historical events.

This viewpoint has been shared by a number of social scientists (Hammersley, 1992; Ackroyd and Hughes, 1992; Bryman, 1992), who were keen to deconstruct the divide between qualitative and quantitative approaches. Hammersley (1992, p.182), cautioned that such a divide 'misrepresents the basis on which decisions should be made' and that 'what is involved is not a cross-roads where we have to go left or right. A better analogy is a complex maze where we are repeatedly faced with decisions, and where paths wind back on one another.' Hammersley further argues that the case study should be viewed as one of many case selection strategies.

While this questioning of the divide between methodologies and theoretical perspectives is healthy, using multiple methodological approaches and analysing multiple forms of data (as in case studies) is far from simple.

However, there are also benefits. The case study approach not only influences the questions to be posed but also allows for how and why questions. It is therefore particularly useful in studies on contemporary phenomena, in which the investigator has little or no control over the course of events. The major strength of the case study approach is that it allows an investigation to retain the holistic nature and complexities of a phenomenon, providing at the same time a systematic inquiry and understanding of particulars.

So the case study approach was selected as the most appropriate method and the case was defined as 'the experiences of a patient facing impending death and those of the nurse(s) who care for him/her'. Participant observation and interviews were selected as the principal methods for collecting data.

Analytical versus statistical generalisation in the conduct of case studies

So far the discussion has dealt with case studies in a general sense, but it is important to consider the question of how to conduct and interpret studies in which multiple cases are included. Yin (1989, p.38) distinguishes between the use of the 'analytical generalisation' and 'statistical generalisation'. For instance, analysing multiple case studies is not the same as analysing multiple respondents in a survey or multiple subjects in an experiment. In the latter, there is an attempt to gain information about a large population from a sample, an approach that is appropriate where simple quantitative questions are to be examined (such as the change in a demographic measurement over time). However, the large number of variables inherent in a study of social phenomena, such as patients' experiences of dying, makes a design involving sampling logic quite inappropriate. As Yin (1989, p.55) states: 'This would require an impossibly large number of cases — too large to allow any statistical consideration of the relevant variables.' Instead, it is more appropriate to consider each individual case as a 'whole study' in its own right. In other words, multiple case studies do not determine prevalence or frequency of a particular phenomenon, but rather they serve to provide compelling support for propositions related to a particular topic. Expounding on this issue, Mitchell (1983, p.207) stated that within the case study approach 'the validity of the extrapolation depends not on the typicality or representativeness of the case but upon the cogency of the theoretical reasoning'.

My study design therefore followed the guiding principle of analytical generalisation as applied to multiple case studies (Mitchell, 1983; Yin, 1989). This meant that typical criteria for selecting a sample, such as the number of cases that can represent, in statistical terms, a larger pool of the population, did not apply. In addition, unlike surveys and experimental studies where the use of probability theory and statistical techniques are needed to generalise from samples to finite populations, the 'populations' of studies (including this one) that are concerned with past, present and future instances to which particular theories claim to apply are infinite. In such situations, where developing and testing theories is concerned, the issue of probability sampling has been viewed as inapplicable to the problem of selecting cases for study (Hammersley, 1992; Mitchell, 1983; Znaniecki, 1934).

In conclusion, therefore, the use of case studies is a generally accepted method for recording and analysing complex information pertaining to social phenomena and would therefore appear to be an appropriate means for investigating the experiences of dying patients and of the nurses caring for them. A multiple case study design such as this one does not raise questions of sampling logic (how many cases should be included to reach statistical significance), since quantitative conclusions are not sought.

Theoretical approach taken in analysing data

The analysis of the cases followed the 'interpretive' perspective (Denzin, 1989b) in contrast to a 'positivistic' model. It sought to uncover, make accessible and reveal the meanings that are used by patients and nurses to make sense of their daily lives in the hospice. In this way, the study attempted to answer 'what' and 'how' questions, rather than 'why' questions about death and dying. That is, the study was not concerned with establishing causal connections but, rather, to describe and interpret the subjective human experiences of death and dying.

Appendix 2: General approach and research strategies in this study

The study was conducted over four years and located in my own practice area. The first year involved spending time in formulating and refining the proposed area of work. By using my experience in practice and a review of the methods used in this particular field of research, discussions and critiques of particular approaches took place with my supervisor and advisers. Initially it appeared that the work could be divided neatly into two phases — the first focusing on experiences of patients and the second on the nurses' responses. However, in reality, the relationships and experiences of both patients and nurses were intertwined and, therefore, to divide them would have created a false separation. Consequently, each case study contains both the patient's and the key nurses' experiences.

Conducting research on dying people tends to evoke a mixture of responses, and a conscious decision was taken at the outset to consider the moral implications of the work. As part of this, the strategy included a system of 'constant challenges' on my motivation, as well as clarifying and pre-empting areas where conflicts of interest might appear. This was conducted by keeping a personal reflective diary, field notes and discussions with my supervisor and colleagues in practice. A mechanism for support was acknowledged at the outset of the study and built in as a vital part of its methodology. An account of the support required and the impact of this study on me is described in the postscript.

ETHICAL CONSIDERATIONS

The research proposal was approved by the health authority's ethics committee. However, in this type of study, ethical and moral considerations do not end on receiving a letter of approval.

Dying people, whether older people or children, are perceived by society as vulnerable groups, and the subject of dying has always been emotive and sensitive (Farberow, 1963; Lee, 1993). This leads some to the view that it is morally unjustifiable to involve dying people in research (De Raeve, 1994). Lee (1993) highlighted the difficulties confronting researchers who study such sensitive topics. These include methodological and technical problems, potential emotional and psychological costs to those involved (including the researcher), and broader issues, such as ethics, politics and legality.

In considering whether it is justifiable to involve dying people in research studies, it is important to look closely at the definition of dying people in this particular study. In the clinical environment where I conducted my research, patients' dying trajectories varied from weeks to months and even to years. So, although a group of such patients may be perceived as dying, in so far as they face certain death at an uncertain time in the future, for many of them there was still a lot of living to do.

The central issues here are fundamentally about how we perceive and behave towards dying people. One view is that dying people are in need of protection and should not be approached for research. An alternative view is that everyone, whether dying or not, should make the choice for themselves (Mount, Cohen, McDonald et al, 1995). The former view has paternalistic overtones — not only does it remove choice, decision-making and thus autonomy from patients, but it also inadvertently introduces an element of discrimination against them. In contrast, the pro-choice viewpoint, although avoiding the danger of paternalism, is potentially open to misuse. In order to make appropriate decisions, patients must be fully informed of the advantages and disadvantages of being involved. They must retain the right to withdraw at any time without care being compromised. Adopting the pro-choice viewpoint inevitably places difficulties in the path of the researcher. For instance, some patients may choose not to exercise a choice, and it then becomes especially important for the researcher to exercise integrity and respect with regard to their best interests. The researcher must at all times guard against abuse of professional power through blinkered pursuit of the research goal and must constantly evaluate the patient's condition and whether he or she still wishes to participate.

On balance, it appeared to me that the crux of the debate is how dying people are viewed and treated *per se*. Clearly, it would be difficult to defend the paternalistic approach when patients are fully aware and competent. I therefore decided that, providing they were mentally competent and fully aware of what was involved, patients should have the right to make decisions for themselves. The process and outcomes of the research were fully explained, their wishes were respected and sensitivity was exercised at all times with respect to their needs as people requiring medical and nursing care.

LOCATION OF FIELDWORK

The research was carried out in an NHS-funded hospice in a provincial teaching hospital. Patients referred there for palliative care usually have a limited life expectancy. Most are diagnosed as having advanced cancer. The main aim of the service is centred on supporting patients at home as far as possible. The hospice provides three primary services: in-patient care, day centre support and home care.

In-patient care

The in-patient unit has 20 beds. In-patients and their families often require support in physical care (including medical and nursing management of symptom control and pain relief), psychosocial care, respite care and terminal care. The process from referral to admission varies between patients. Most are initially seen at out-patient clinics, some during domiciliary visits, and others in the in-patient unit (such as when they arrive by ambulance as emergency admissions). The latter group is often very ill and their deaths may be imminent. In recent years the profile of patients admitted has shifted towards an acute model of hospice care. Admission is increasingly aimed at preventing and dissipating crisis from occurring at home. Thus, patients who are admitted usually require immediate management. On average, most patients spend about 10 days as an in-patient during an admission, with the emphasis focused on stabilising their condition so that they can be supported at home. Approximately 50% of the hospice patients die in the in-patient unit, 30% die at home and 15% in other hospitals.

Three teams of nurses operate during the day. At night, a team of nurses oversees the care of all patients in the three teams. Patients are assigned to a specific team of day nurses on admission. Most patients present with multiple problems which may be primarily physical, associated with advanced malignancies or with family dynamics and functioning. Often the nursing work is labour-intensive and emotionally and physically heavy. Consequently, it is not unusual to find the in-patient unit resembling a busy acute medical ward, as opposed to a calm, peaceful, quiet setting as envisioned in the ideal hospice environment espoused by traditional hospice rhetoric (Walter, 1994).

Day centre

The day centre operates from Monday until Friday. Patients arrive from 10am and return home at 3.30pm. The centre serves two functions — to provide a focal point where patients can meet for support through social and therapeutic activities and as a monitoring service. The day-centre activities operate at different levels and include general chit-chat, participating in quizzes, preparing goods for sale at bazaars, watching invited performances (such as the Royal Ballet and Irish dancing), music therapy, support groups, massage and expression of feelings through poems and prose. Patients using this service are normally referred via out-patients, or from the in-patient unit following discharge home. Each of the four nurses working in the day centre has her own caseload. Each group of patients uses the day centre on an assigned day of the week. An individual patient's progress (and family situation) are reviewed by the patient's assigned nurse, and any deterioration or problems are assessed jointly by the mutidisciplinary team. Most patients attending the day centre are able to maintain a fair amount of independence. The centre acts as a support to patients and their families by creating space and providing both parties with an opportunity for personal time. It is, in effect, a halfway house, bridging the care provided at home and by professionals. In contrast to the in-patient unit, the busy nature of the day centre takes the form of a relaxed, noisy, lively hubbub of human activities

Home care

As the overall aim of the hospice is to support patients at home, the home care service is an integral component of the patients' total care. This service has expanded in the past decade and is provided by a team of five Macmillan nurses. This title reflects the initial source of funding for establishing these posts, the Macmillan Cancer Relief Fund. Each Macmillan nurse has her own caseload of about 16 patients and meets new patients through attendance with the consultant physicians at various clinical settings. The Macmillan nurses, therefore, have diverse roles: to advocate for patients, to assess physical and family situations and implement management of care as required, and to liaise between the hospice and primary health care team in the community.

Most patients use all three hospice care services during their admission. For instance, patients who have been in-patients also use the home care service, either being referred by the Macmillan nurse for admission initially or being referred by the in-patient nurses to the Macmillan nurses on discharge home. Similarly, patients who use the day centre are often allocated to a Macmillan nurse. On the whole, continuity of care for patients throughout the three areas is maintained by formal and informal interaction between the nurses and other health care professionals.

NEGOTIATING ACCESS AND WORKING ARRANGEMENTS

During the planning of the research, negotiations for support of the study took place, initially with the senior nurse and medical colleagues and subsequently with the rest of my nursing colleagues at the sisters' meeting. My interest in pursuing the study was generally well received. One concern related to the timing for approaching patients to participate in the study. For instance, new patients arriving in out-patients or the hospice for the first time have a great deal of new information and experiences with which to cope. It was felt that they should not be burdened by an additional request to participate in research, particularly in view of its topic. Admission to hospital increases anxieties (Cartwright, 1964; Duff and Hollingshead, 1968; Franklin, 1974), and this can be expected to be magnified in hospices which, for some people, conjure an image of the 'death house'. This view is often expressed to me by neighbours, taxi drivers and friends when they discover where I work. The issue of when and how to approach patients was therefore important. Clearly, sensitivity, tact and timing were crucial in order not to jeopardise the confidence, trust and future care of potential participants in the study.

Following a general review of the three service areas in conjunction with the senior nurse, it appeared that the best area in which to approach patients for the study was via the day centre.

This decision was taken for the following reasons:

- Generally, patients in the day centre were fairly well and therefore there was time for me to foster and build relationships with the patients before they became less well. This also allowed time for newly referred patients to settle and get used to the hospice before being approached

- Patients use the day centre partly for social reasons, and conversations with staff and other patients form a normal part of the day's activities

- Some patients attending the day centre already had experience of in-patient or home care. They were therefore used to the hospice and the care delivered

- Patients referred to the day centre were likely to use the in-patient and home care services at some time. I would therefore be able to obtain an all-round view of dying and death in different settings. Recruiting patients from the day centre did not preclude being able to observe and follow patients in the other settings.

The second level of negotiation involved the day centre sister, who agreed in the first instance to approach a few patients whom she knew would 'enjoy talking' to see if they would like to participate in the research as a 'first run'.

My practice area at the start of the study was in the in-patient unit — I was doing blocks of two weeks' practice, usually out of term time. However, during the second year of the study I negotiated for the practice component of my job as lecturer–practitioner to be based at the day centre. This enabled me to become immersed in the profiles of patients in the day centre as well as being able to get a sense of what was happening to the patients. Thus, I was able to note both subtle and formal developments of events.

SELECTION OF PATIENTS FOR CASE STUDIES

The demographic data of all patients admitted for terminal care between 1989 and 1993 were scrutinised for the percentage of male and female referrals, primary cancer sites and age range. Purposive sampling was employed (Robson, 1993). The aim was for the cases to reflect, as closely as possible factors that may be of significance during the dying trajectory — for instance, age, time elements, gender, home support, and the primary cancer site — and the main dimensions and characteristics of the hospice population. Table 3 shows the age, sex, marital status, and primary cancer sites of patients selected. Table 4 provides a comparison between the cases and the general experience of the hospice, from which the cases were drawn. The cases show a broadly similar sex distribution (women in the majority) and age predominance (mean age close to 60) to the general hospice population. Carcinoma of the breast was the commonest primary tumour, as in the hospice population. Therefore, the cases can be seen to reflect some of the key characteristics of the hospice population as a whole.

Table 3. Demographic data for the selected cases (patients)

Case	Sex	Age	Primary cancer site	Marital status
1	F	46	breast	married
2	F	60	breast	widow
3	F	60	breast	married
4	M	50	testis	married
5	F	44	breast	divorced
6	F	35	glioma	single
7	F	70	breast	divorced
8	F	70	lung	divorced
9	M	67	colorectal	married
10	M	82	colorectal	married
11	M	67	prostate	married
12	M	48	colorectal	married

Table 4. Comparison of demographic data between selected cases (patients) and hospice population

	N	Mean Age (range)	% Male	% Female	% Patients with primary tumour in: Breast	Colo-rectal	Lung	Prostate	Glioma	Testis
Cases (1991–94)*	12	58.3 (35-82)	41.6	58.4	41.6	25.0	8.3	8.3	8.3	8.3
Hospice (1989–93)*	1927	66.9	48.4	51.6	24.0	10.0	16.0	7.0	2.0	0.2

* Case studied between 1991 and 1994. Hospice data based on statistics collected between 1989 and 1993. 1994-onwards: data not available at time of study.

Twelve cases were chosen for inclusion. Seven were women patients and their nurses, and five were men and their nurses. A total of 15 nurses were interviewed (there was more than one nurse per patient), two men and 13 women. The nurses' ages ranged between 25 and 52 years.

CRITERIA FOR APPROACHING PARTICIPANTS (PATIENTS AND NURSES) FOR THE STUDY

Treating individuals as a means to a research goal can potentially conflict with their interests. In my study patients were present because they required care, and therefore the care element was primary and took precedence over the research. Patients facing imminent death on admission were not approached to participate. Instead, I approached only those who were fully aware, willing to participate and who had settled into the routine of hospice care. I also checked carefully with patients and their nurse that my time with them was not compromising their treatment or other activities.

The criteria for patient inclusion were:

- aged 18 years and older;
- admitted during the study period for palliative care;
- fully conscious and aware;
- able to communicate in English;
- willing to participate.

Nurses who were assigned to the care of the patient during the study period were approached to participate in the study, provided they were willing to do so.

METHOD OF APPROACHING PATIENTS AND NURSES

Data collection began in March 1991 and was completed in March 1994. The initial group of four patients and their nurses constituted the 'first run' of the study. They comprise Cases 1 to 4 in Table 3. Subsequently I found that it was realistic to have no more than four to five patients at any one time so, when a patient died, I was able to approach another to participate in the study. When approaching patients I would introduce myself and explain about the study, the methods of collecting data and the reasons for conducting the work. In general, the response was supportive and positive. At this meeting I also emphasised that participants were free to withdraw at any time without prejudice to themselves. I stressed that the interview tapes were confidential and that the recordings would be erased when the study was completed. Following this initial meeting I would return the following week to check whether the person wished to be included in the study. Most were keen and asked when we would begin the first interview — this usually happened on the same day. Over the three-year period 12 patients agreed to participate and three declined. As the research involves following patients prospectively, it was decided to implement a system of 'process consenting' (Munhall, 1988), in which continual checks were made at intervals to establish whether the patient still wished to participate. No one withdrew. Similarly, nurses' willingness to participate was also checked at intervals and the general principles outlined for approaching patients were also applied to nurses. All nurses approached agreed to participate and none withdrew.

COLLECTION OF DATA

Multiple sources of data collection were used. These included a combination of approaches: observations arising directly from my role as participant observer, regular informal interviews with patients and nurses, nursing and medical documentation and materials such as poems, prose or music composed by patients. A field diary recording my interactions, thoughts and feelings was also kept. Case profiles were gradually generated for each patient and their nurse(s). As participant observation and interviews were the main data collection strategies, they are described in detail below.

Participant observation and interviews

The advantages and limitations of using participant observation as a method have been thoroughly discussed both theoretically (Jorgensen, 1989; Ackroyd and Hughes, 1992) and empirically (Melia, 1981; James, 1986; Samarel, 1991). There appear to be four possible roles open to the participant observer (Gold, 1958; Junker, 1960; Pearsall, 1965), ranging from complete participant to complete observer, with participant-as-observer and observer-as-participant in between. In the participant-as-observer role, both researcher and participants are aware of each others' roles, and close relationships may be developed. In the observer-as-participant role, the researcher remains detached and involvement with subjects is deliberately kept to a minimum. My role in this study was mainly participant-as-observer. I continued to practise as a nurse in the unit, attended meetings and, on occasions, accompanied the Macmillan nurses to the patients' homes. I observed conversations, nurse-patient interactions and relevant nursing and medical documentation that directly pertained to the cases I was studying.

My nursing experience provided me with several advantages as a participant observer: for instance, being accepted and supported by colleagues in the hospice, being at ease with patients and nurses participating and, above all, being able to identify issues pertinent to nursing. Problems that may be experienced by an outsider using participant observation, therefore, did not apply in my case (Jorgensen, 1989; Ackroyd and Hughes, 1992). However, there were other issues that I had to consider as an insider. For instance, having inside knowledge meant that I was not a naïve observer, and there was always the potential risk of jumping to preconceived conclusions about events. I was therefore conscious of the need to keep an open mind. Another concern related to potential conflicts of interest regarding my role as both a nurse and a researcher in a clinical area where I also held a senior nursing position. I felt it was important to clarify my role during the period of the study, particularly when I was caring for the patients. For instance, depending on whether I was viewed as a nurse or researcher, patients' disclosure of their situations and how the information disclosed is subsequently used could have had potential moral implications.

I did not automatically assume that information given to me by patients while I was acting as their nurse should be used in the study. When patients in the study were assigned to me to look after, I would explain to them that I was working as their nurse that day. Sometimes, the patients would share new information about their progress. If this appeared relevant to the research, I would ask permission to include it in the study.

Direct and indirect observations made during the day were recorded in my field diary. However, as the focus of the study was to gain an understanding of the patients' and nurses' experiences, it was important that information was gathered directly from the participants themselves. Informal, focused interviews formed a crucial component of this study.

Location and frequency of interviews

Interviews with patients and nurses were conducted individually in a quiet room, by patients' bedsides in the in-patient unit or in the patients' own homes. Each interview lasted about 20-30 minutes and was repeated with a frequency that varied depending on the pace, depth and content of each case. For instance, it would usually take three interviews to reach deep into a subject or experience, whereas for a few patients, rich and deep accounts were elicited during the first interview. In between interviews I would attend staff meetings to get feedback on patients' progress and, in particular, to make notes on any significant changes in their conditions. Whenever there were indications of significant developments I tried to interview the patients and nurses involved to find out their response. The nurse interviews were easily forthcoming, with a considerable amount of personal reflection and insights. These took place at work when it was convenient for the nurse to meet with me. Table 5 summarises the length of my contact with the patients, the place of death and the number of conversations conducted with them, and their nurses.

Table 5. Details of contact and place of death for selected cases

Number of conversations with:

Case number	Contact (months)	Patient	Nurse	Place of death
1	6	6	5	Hospice
2	14	12	10	Hospice
3	7	6	5	Home
4	38	15	16	Living
5	18	12	10	Hospice
6	20	15	10	Hospice
7	18	9	8	Living
8	17	6	6	Living
9	4	5	7	Acute hospital
10	8	6	5	Hospice
11	2	4	4	Hospice
12	6	6	6	Hospice

RECORDING OF INTERVIEWS AND OTHER DATA

Each encounter with patients and nurses was recorded in a field diary. I also jotted down the context of these encounters to avoid losing the ambience of the atmosphere and scenes as I perceived them at the time. I also wrote analytical memos to myself, and these served as the backdrop and guide during the periods of data analysis. I used a small dictaphone in the interviews and most patients did not object to having their conversations recorded, except for one who once requested that I write it down.

STRATEGY AND CONTENT OF INTERVIEWS

An informal, conversational, 'funnel' approach (Denzin, 1978) was used in interview. This method provided opportunities to probe, clarify and explore issues as they occurred. The conversations I held with patients centred around three key areas:

- feelings and reactions about dying;

- experiences before and during the living-dying phase;

- wishes and thoughts about the manner of death when it occurs.

These three themes enabled me to uncover what Feigenberg (1980) described as the three governing elements of any individual's life. That is, during life there is always a present, a past and a future. According to Feigenberg (1980, p.12), the dying person's existence consists of what is happening now (dying), what has happened (life up to now) and what is going to happen (death and that which comes after death, however this may be conceived). During the first interview I used an opening phrase such as: 'Could you tell me a bit about yourself and your illness since the time of your diagnosis?' to initiate the conversation. As time went on, in subsequent interviews I would use phrases such as: 'Tell me how you feel and what's been happening to you since we last met' or 'How do you see the future?' Significant events or developments were followed and raised for exploration with the patients during the interviews.

Conversations with the nurses were focused primarily on their responses to the experiences and expressions of patients' dying. The conversations focused on the following areas:

- nurses' perceptions of patients' experiences: for instance, patients' progress and expressions of their dying;

- issues that were particularly difficult or satisfying, or about which the nurse was ambivalent, in the care of that particular patient;

- responses and actions in relation to the experiences and expressions of patients in nursing practice.

Closure of interviewing sessions and of the interview process

It was inevitable that sometimes patients and nurses were sad when talking about their experiences. On other occasions, however, feelings of joy and happiness were also expressed. In the former situation I would check to see whether the interviewee wanted to carry on talking. It was also important that they were not left at the end of the interview without knowing that further support was available, if necessary. Consequently, an important aspect of closure was for me to be honest and to ask the patient whether they would like me to tell their nurse what had happened. This offer was sometimes taken up. Similarly, with the nurses I would equally check to make sure that they were not left feeling unsupported.

There came a time in the course of interviewing when it became clear that there might not be an opportunity to meet up with the patients again, especially when physical deterioration was evident. I would use such occasions to thank the patients for their help with acknowledging the closure of that aspect of my relationship with them. I found this to be an important act for me, albeit a sad one. In some cases the patients had been participating in the study for almost two years, and during that time my feelings and respect for them had deepened.

V: Postscript, references and index

Postscript

During the course of undertaking this research, my colleagues and other doctoral students often asked how I managed to cope with the emotional exposure demanded by a prospective study of death and dying. In particular, they sought an understanding the effects of exposure to the emotional aspects of the work and strategies for coping with it long term. I agreed that it was emotionally hard work, even though I had previous experience of nursing the dying and therefore knew something of what to expect in a hospice. I also tried hard to explain the different emotional involvement between being a nurse caring, and a research student. I shall therefore discuss this aspect of the research methodology in the hope that it will prove helpful to those embarking on similar work.

In any study that aims to gain meaningful insight into experiences as they occur there is clearly the need to establish a relationship of trust and respect with the participants. However, the nature of my work meant that the initial relationship often developed and became deeper with time. The relationship I developed with the patients differed from a typical nurse-patient relationship, with its focus on professional care, because I was asking them to provide me with an account of their feelings, thoughts and actions in order to enable me understand those experiences.

Moreover, unlike everyday nursing, where it is normally possible to 'switch off' after work, or 'let go' of the patients after they have died (and, in so doing, move on to new patients and situations), in the research I found myself having to resurrect the patients who had died, and relive and re-engage in their experiences weeks and months later. Often this involved listening to their voices from the tape-recordings and reading their experiences on transcripts, and I found this emotionally extremely hard going.

Several times, during periods of intense data analysis, I found that my thoughts were stimulated to the extent that I could see the faces of the patients who had died. I dreamt about them and sensed their presence. They became, once again, alive and real. These experiences were rather spooky for me. Such occurrences, I discovered subsequently, were not unusual, as demonstrated by Qvarnstrom's (1978) and McLean's (1993) accounts of undertaking research work with dying people. For instance, Qvarnstrom (1978, p.161) wrote: 'After a patient's death, I would relive his dying process on the subconscious level. In dreams, the patient's whole pathology, dying moment and state of being dead would be rehearsed anew. As a dead person in my dreams the patient went through different states of existence, ranging from the human appearance that was delineated at the moment of death to the skeleton's decomposition into bones.'

More recently, in her work with leukaemia patients, McLean (1993, p.205) stated: '...from my perspective, the research method had an emotional cost. In choosing to explore the experience of leukaemia, I encountered and became involved with people in crisis. In order to cope with the emotional stresses associated with the intense personal involvement, I adopted various coping strategies...'

Fortunately, I realised the need for personal support at the outset of the study and built it in as a vital part of the methodology. Formal and informal support was provided at different times throughout the four years of the project. One of the most useful aspects of this support comprised formal supervision counselling sessions during key times in the study. These were negotiated on a regular basis and centred around the times of data analysis.

With the help of my counsellor I was able to make some sense of my experiences. For instance, my counsellor would explain that, having asked the patients for their experiences, it was not inconceivable that I should carry their 'ghosts' at certain times. Projections of part of the patients' selves may have had an influence on me and that may be why I perceived them as alive. Strong emotions were off-loaded on to me during interviews, and these could also be present (particularly with patients that I had grown to like or formed stronger bonds with). Moreover, like the nurses and patients in the study, I also watched and waited as patients deteriorated and progressive losses became evident. Listening at first hand to the patients' expressions of profound distress and sadness at their losses, and constant searching for their meanings, was an emotionally draining experience. My counsellor and I agreed that I should write notes following our sessions together, in order to monitor any progress, and to provide written documentation that could be used later to illuminate the emotional impact of the research. Here are two extracts from my personal diary that traced my progress:

October 20, 1993

Saw Mary for my first session of supervision counselling on my PhD work. Finding it emotionally difficult to do my analyses. I kept seeing the patients' faces and feeling sad. Mary runs stress management courses for health care professionals and appears spot-on in her ability to cue in on key issues in my work.

Key issues raised

GC: Two key times when the work gets to me:

a)   when patients die;

b)   during analyses of data when I get spooked.

Mary pointed out that the stress of the work appears to be from two fronts:

a)   the PhD itself;

b)   the nature of relationships established with patients in the study.

Mary highlighted the following pertinent points:

I asked the patients for their experiences and as a consequence they volunteer and I carry their ghosts, as it were. Mary talked about projections of part of their selves as having an influence on me and said it might be useful to explore this element a bit deeper in subsequent sessions, if I agreed.

Mary also helped me distinguish between this work and nursing of dying patients generally.

In the PhD, I establish a relationship with patients to get the data and patients possibly use me to offload.

However, unlike normal nursing, where one lets go when a patient dies, as the researcher I ask for the information and, moreover, have to resurrect them months later to relive their experiences. That's when they come alive for me. Some strong emotions that have been offloaded to me may still be present — also have impact in data analyses selection of data and focus?

Mary also asked me whether I have been listening to their voices on the tapes during analyses. That was a good question because to date I have found that difficult... have I been trying to avoid that??!! I said that would have to come and perhaps I am pacing myself for when I shall be ready. I remember one of the patients was about to die when I wrote the report and two others had recently died together. Tapes, transcripts all seemed to mesh together.

October 24, 1993

Second session with Mary. Today we explored a bit deeper how I was feeling. I told Mary that since our first session I have been able to feel more at ease with the current period of analysis. For example, I have listened to the tapes of my conversations with patients who have died and I am more at ease with that. I have had one or two dreams about them but have not felt so spooked. For instance, I feel OK even if I should feel that their spirits are around me. That is alright, too, for at least I can make sense of what may be happening in this work. I talked about the poignancy of Peter's last days and also about what I was still feeling about Susan, despite the fact that she died around two years ago. What was operating there? I talked about her death and dying and perhaps identifying with her. For example, someone with young children, and the relationship with her sister which has never been fostered, comparing to my own situation of having a sister who is so far away. And thinking: would it be similar for me if I were in Susan's position? We then compared this case with Peter's. Peter's case was different; he was a man, albeit with a young child. However, the situation with Peter was also different because he was trying to impart this 'gift', as it were, which was his very personal experience of what he was going through as he lay dying; that is, what was dying like for him and hoping I could capture it?

The key things we discussed were:

- *Am I acting as an auxiliary ego for these patients?*

- *Have I taken on a 'godmother/aunt' role that they could share these rather specific things with, knowing that I am interested in dying, as opposed to the 'mother' role of their nurses, who perhaps take on other duties as well, such as medicines etc?*

- *Am I also acting as a marker for them in terms of their dying? That is, as they talk, is it also helping them articulate and making it more explicit in terms of where they are with themselves?*

We also discussed the notion of patients' dignity — Mary talked in terms of being able to maintain adult dignity — the notion of OK, even if things appear terrible to others around, dignity [is] still maintained if [the] degree and level of terrible pain is OK with that patient. An example is a woman screaming at childbirth — acceptable for the woman and the midwife if that expression facilitates the birth and likewise with dying (a particular patient I nursed ages ago, despite drugs, still screamed at death). Question: Is it so that for a small minority that is how dying would be expressed? Can death and dying ever be dignified?

I felt that in this session I am more at ease now, in terms of understanding in greater depth the issues that may operate, those that overlap and conflict with me as a nurse and researcher. I feel also there is a light at the end of the tunnel and I talked to Mary of the relief I would feel when the thesis is complete and I can release all these ghosts — that is, go to the top of a hill, erase all these tapes and let them all go. Wow! We arranged to meet in January 1994.

Working closely both with the patients and nurses, therefore, demanded considerable emotional effort on my part during the course of this study. A major element of the work was to remain in touch and stay with events as they unfolded. While this had many strengths in terms of the grounding of the study, it is clear that it also carried a major disadvantage. This is probably best summed up as a 'triple-layered' phenomenon. In the first instance, I was directly exposed to the patients' accounts of their sadness associated with progressive losses; in the second, I was equally exposed to the emotions and feelings expressed by the nurses; and in the third, I experienced my own feelings of loss when patients in the study died. For instance, when this happened, I found myself experiencing a range of emotions: sadness, anger and relief, often in a haphazard fashion. Moreover, it was especially difficult when the timing of the patient's death was unexpected. This occurred particularly with Alan (case 10). On reflection, the lack of opportunity to thank him for his contribution to the research and to say goodbye (thus constituting a closure) was particularly sad. It may well reflect my own needs as an individual. I also found I needed to talk about my feelings in those instances.

As well as the formal supervision counselling sessions, the other strategies of support included building on the mechanisms that I was already using personally and professionally. These included time out for holidays, spending time with my family and friends, swimming, gardening and being able to acknowledge my own feelings openly to myself as well as sharing, in confidence, how I felt with my supervisor and colleagues. This support was always a tremendous help and a vital balance, and without it I would have found it difficult to pursue research of this nature in any depth. Finally, and paradoxically, the patients' courage, sense of humour and encouragement provided me with the help and resolve to continue with the work.

References

Abel, E.K (1986) The hospice movement: Institutionalizing innovation. *International Journal of Health Services*; 16: 1, 71–85.

Ackroyd, S & Hughes, J. (1992) *Data Collection in Context.* London: Longman.

Addington–Hall, J.M., MacDonald, L.D., Anderson, H.R. (1990) Can the Spitzer Quality of Life Index help to reduce prognostic uncertainty in terminal care? *British Journal of Cancer*; 62: 695–699.

Aldrich, C.K. (1963) The dying patient's grief. *Journal of American Medical Association*; 184: 329–331.

Alexander, D.A., Ritchie, E. (1990) Stressors and difficulties in dealing with the terminal patient. *Journal of Palliative Care*; 6: 3, 28–33.

Alexander, M. (1980) The rigid embrace of the narrow house: Premature burial and the signs of death. *Hastings Centre Report*; June 10, 25–31.

Amenta, M.M. (1984) Traits of hospice nurses compared with those who work in traditional settings. *Journal of Clinical Psychology*; 40: 2, 414–420.

Aries, P. (1983) *Western Attitudes Towards Death.* Baltimore: John Hopkins University Press.

Armstrong, D. (1983) The fabrication of nurse–patient relationships. *Social Science and Medicine*; 17: 8, 457–460.

Armstrong, D. (1987) Silence and truth in death and dying. *Social Science and Medicine*; 24: 8, 651–657.

Back, I.N. (1992) Terminal restlessness in patients with advanced malignant disease. *Palliative Medicine*; 6: 4, 293–298.

Backer, B.A., Hannon, N., Russell, N.A. (1982) *Death and Dying: Individuals and Institutions*. New York: John Wiley and Sons.

Barraclough, J. (1994) *Cancer and Emotion*. New York: John Wiley & Sons.

Becker, E. (1973) *The Denial of Death*. New York: Free Press.

Benner, P. (1984) *From Novice to Expert: Excellence and power in clinical nursing practice*. Menlo Park, California: Addison–Wesley.

Benner, P. (1985) The oncology clinical nursing specialist: an expert coach. *Oncology Nursing Forum*; 12: 2, 40.

Benner, P., Wrubel, J. (1989) *The Primacy of Caring*. Menlo Park, California: Addison–Wesley.

Berelson, B. (1971) Cited by Mostyn, B. (1985) The content analysis of qualitative research data: A dynamic approach. In: Brenner, M., Brown, J., Canter, D. (eds). *The Research Interview*. New York: Academic Press.

Bergen, A. (1992) Evaluating nursing care of the terminally ill in the community: a case study approach. *International Journal of Nursing Studies*; 29: 1, 81–94.

Bennum, I. (1988) Systems theory and family therapy. In Street, E., Dryden, W. (eds) *Family Therapy in Britain*. Open University Press.

Bertman, S. L. (1991) *Facing Death: images, insights and interventions*. New York: Hemisphere Publishing Corporation.

Birch, J. (1979) Anxiety and conflict in nurse education. In: Davis, B.D (ed) *Research in Nurse Education*. London: Croom Helm.

Blauner, R. (1966) Death and social structure. *Psychiatry*; 29: 378–394.

Bliss, J., Monk, M., Ugborn, J. (1983) *Qualitative Data Analysis for Educational Research: a guide to uses of systematic networks*. London: Croom Helm.

Blumer, H. (1962) Society as symbolic interaction. In: Rose, A.M. (ed) *Human Behaviour and Social Processes*. Boston: Houghton Mifflin.

Blumer, H. (1969) *Symbolic Interactionism*. New Jersey: Prentice Hall.

Bogdan, R., Biklen, S.K. (1992) *Qualitative Research for Education: an introduction to theory and methods*. (2nd ed). Boston: Allyn & Bacon.

Bowers, M. (1975) *Counselling the Dying*. New York: Jason Aronson.

Bowker, J. (1991) *The Meanings of Death.* New York: Cambridge University Press.

Boyar, J.I. (1964) *The Constriction and Partial Validation of a Scale for the Measurement of the Fear of Death.* PhD. dissertation. New York: University of Rochester.

Bram, P.J., Katz, L. (1989) A study of burnout in nurses working in hospice and hospital oncology settings. *Oncology Nursing Forum;* 16: 4, 555–560.

Brown, L. (1986) The experience of care: patient perspectives. *Topics in Clinical Nursing;* 8: 2, 56–62.

Bryman A (1992) *Quantity and Quality in Social Research.* London: Routledge.

Buckman (1993) Communication in palliative care: a practical guide. In Doyle, D., Hanks, G.W.C., MacDonald, N. (eds). *Oxford Textbook of Palliative Medicine;* Oxford Medical Publications.

Buckmann, R. (1988) *I Don't Know What to Say: how to help and support someone who is dying.* London: Macmillan Publishers.

Burgess R. (1984) *In the Field: an introduction to field research.* London: Unwin Hyman.

Burnham, J., Harris, Q. (1988) Systemic family therapy. In Street, E., Dryden W. (eds). *Family Therapy in Britain.* Milton Keynes: Open University Press.

Burnham, J. (1990) *Family Therapy.* London & New York: Tavistock & Routledge.

Campbell, A.V. (1984) *Moderated love: A Theology of Professional Care.* London: Society for the Promotion of Christian Knowledge.

Cappon, D. (1959) The Dying. *Psychiatric Quarterly;* 33: 466–489.

Cappon, D. (1962) Attitudes of and towards the dying. *Canadian Medical Association Journal;* 87: 693–700.

Carey, R. (1974) Emotional adjustment in terminal patients: A quantitative approach. *Journal of Counselling Psychology;* 21: 5, 433–439.

Carney, T.F. (1990) *Collaborative Inquiry Methodology.* Windsor, Ontario, Canada: University of Windsor. In: Miles, M.B. & Huberman, A.M. (1994) *Qualitative Data Analysis.* London: Sage Publications.

Carter, E., McGoldrick, M. (1980) *The Family Life Cycle.* New York: Gardner.

Cartwright, A. (1964) *Human Relations and Hospital Care.* London: Routledge and Kegan Paul.

Cassell, E.J. (1991) *The Nature of Suffering.* Oxford: Oxford University Press.

Castles, M.R., Murray, R, B. (1979) *Dying In An Institution: nurse/patient perspectives.* New York: Appleton–Century Crofts.

Central Statistical Office (1992) *Social Trends 92.* London: HMSO.

Central Statistical Office (1995) *Social Trends 25.* London: HMSO.

Cerny, T., Blair, V., Anderson, H., Bramwell, V., Thatcher, N. (1987) Pretreatment prognostic factors and scoring system in 407 small cell lung cancer patients. *International Journal of Cancer;* 39: 146–149.

Charles–Edwards, A. (1983) *The Nursing Care of the Dying Patient.* Beaconsfield: Beaconsfield Publishers Ltd.

Charmaz, K. (1980) *The Social Reality of Death: death in contemporary America.* Reading, MA: Addison–Wesley.

Charmaz, K. (1983) Loss of self: a fundamental form of suffering in the chronically ill. *Sociology of Health and Illness;* 5: 20, 169–195.

Choron, J. (1964) *Modern Man and Mortality.* New York: Macmillan.

Christensen, J. (1993) *Nursing Partnership; a model for nursing practice.* London: Churchill Livingstone.

Clark, D. (1993a) *The Future for Palliative Care: issues of policy and practice.* Buckingham/Philadelphia: Open University Press, Ch10.

Clark, D. (1993b) *The Sociology of Death.* Oxford: Blackwell Publishers.

Clark, E.J. (1990) Overview of sociology's contribution to intervention in life–threatening illness, dying loss and grief. In: Clark, E.J., Fritz, J.M., Rieker, P.P. (1990) *Clinical Sociological Perspectives on Illness and Loss: The linkage of theory and practice.* Philadelphia: Charles Press.

Cochrane, J.B, Levy M.R, Fryer, J.E., Oglesby, C.A. (1990) Death anxiety, disclosure behaviours, and attitudes of oncologists towards terminal care. *Omega;* 22: 1–12.

Collet, L., Lester, D. (1969) Fear of death and fear of dying. *Journal of Psychology;* 72: 179–181.

References

Collinson, D. (1992) *Fifty Major Philosophers: a reference guide.* London & New York: Routledge.

Conboy–Hill, S. (1986) Terminal care: their death in your hands. *Professional Nurse*; 2: 2, 51–53.

Cooper, C.L. (1984) *Psychosocial Stress and Cancer.* New York: John Wiley & Sons.

Copp, G., Dunn, V. (1993) Frequent and difficult problems perceived by nurses caring for the dying in community, hospice and acute care settings. *Palliative Medicine*; 7: 1, 19–25.

Copp, G. (1994) Palliative Care Nursing Education — a review of research findings. *Journal of Advanced Nursing*; 19: 3, 552–557.

Copp, G. (1995) *Issues of Loss and Grief (1)* In: Webber, J., Dicks, B. (eds), *Issues in Palliative Nursing.* Beaconsfield: Beaconsfield Publishers Ltd.

Corbin J. (1986) *Coding, writing memos and diagramming.* In: Chenitz, W.C., Swanson, J.M. (eds). From Practice to Grounded Theory. Menlo Park, California: Addison–Wellesley.

Corner, J. (1993) *The nursing perspective.* In: Doyle, D., Hanks, G.W.C.. & MacDonald, N. (eds) Oxford Textbook of Palliative Medicine; Oxford: Oxford Medical Publications.

Corr, C.A. (1993) Death in a modern society. In: Doyle, D., Hanks, G.W.C., MacDonald, N. (eds) *Oxford Textbook of Palliative Medicine*; Oxford: Oxford Medical Publications.

Corr, C.A. (1992) A task–based approach to coping with dying. *Omega*; 24: 2, 81–94.

Couch, C.J., Stanley, L., Michael, A. (1986) *Studies in Symbolic Interaction: the Iowa School.* Parts A & B. Greenwich, Conn: JAI Press.

Cox, G., Fundis, R. (1990) Teaching the sociology of dying and death. In Clark, E.J, Fritz, J.M., Rieker, P. (eds). *Clinical Sociological Perspectives on Illness & Loss.* Philadelphia: Charles Press.

Cronin, S.N., Harrison, B. (1988) Importance of nursing caring behaviours as perceived by patients after myocardial infarction. *Heart & Lung*; 17: 4, 374–380.

Csordas, T.J. (1994) *Embodiment and Experience: the existential ground of culture and self.* Cambridge: Cambridge University Press.

Cullberg, J. (1970) and (1971) cited by Qvarnstrom, U. (1978) *Patients Reactions to Impending death.* Stockholm: Stockholm Institute of International Education & Department of Medicine.

Cumming, E., Henry W.E. (1961) *Growing Old: The process of disengagement.* New York: Charles Press.

Davis, B., Oberle, K. (1990) Dimensions of the supportive role of the nurse in palliative care. *Oncology Nursing Forum;* 17: 1, 87–94.

Davis, R. (1973) Organic factors and psychological adjustment in advanced cancer patients. *Psychosomatic Medicine;* 35: 6, 467–471.

De Raeve, L. (1994) Ethical issues in palliative care research. *Palliative Medicine;* 8: 4, 298–305.

Degner, L. (1974) The relationship between some beliefs held by physicians and their life prolonging decisions. *Omega;* 5: 223.

Denzin, N.K. (1978) *The Research Act.* New York: McGraw–Hill.

Denzin, N. (1989a) Interpretive Biography. Newbury Park, California: Sage Publications.

Denzin, N. (1989b) *Interpretive Interactionism.* London: Sage Publications.

Denzin, N. (1992) *Symbolic Interactionism and Cultural Studies: the politics of interpretation.* Oxford: Blackwell Publishers.

Department of Health (1989) *Working for Patients: National Health Service review: Working Paper 2. Funding and contracts for hospital services.* London: HMSO.

Dewey, J. (1896) The Reflex Arc Concept in Psychology. *Psychological Review;* 3: 357–370.

DeWys, W.D., Begg, D., Lavin, P.T. (1980) Prognostic effect of weight loss prior to chemotherapy in cancer patients. *American Journal of Medicine;* 69: 491–499.

Diggory, J.C., Rothman, D.Z. (1961) Values destroyed by death. *Journal of Abnormal and Social Psychology;* 63: 205–210.

Dijkstra,W., Van der Veen, L., Van Der Zouwen, J. (1985) A field experiment on interviewer–respondent interaction. In: Brenner, M., Brown, J., Canter, D. (eds). *The Research Interview.* Academic Press.

Douglas, C. (1992) For all the saints. *British Medical Journal;* 304: 579.

Duclow, D. (1981) *Dying on Broadway: Contemporary drama and mortality.* Soundings. 64, p2.

Duff, R.S., Hollingshead, A.B. (1968) *Sickness and Society.* New York: Harper and Row.

Duke, S., Copp, G. (1992) Hidden nursing in palliative care. *Nursing Times;* 88: 17, 40–42.

Dumont, R.G., Foss, D.C. (1972) *The American View of Death: Acceptance or denial?* Cambridge, Massachussetts: Schenkman.

Dunlop, M.J. (1986) Is a science of caring possible? *Journal of Advanced Nursing;* 11: 6, 661–670.

Elias, N. (1985) *The Loneliness of the Dying.* Oxford: Blackwell Publishers.

Ersser, S. (1992) A search for the therapeutic dimension of nurse–patient interactions. In: McMahon, R., Pearson, A. (eds). *Nursing as a Therapy* London: Chapman and Hall.

Farberow, N. L. (1963) Introduction. In Farberow, N.L. (ed). *Taboo Topics.* New York: Atherton Press.

Farncombe, M., Chater, S. (1993) Case studies outlining use of nebulised morphine for patients with end–stage chronic lung and cardiac disease. *Journal of Pain and Symptom Management;* 8: 4, 221–225.

Feifel, H. (1973) Death fear in dying heart and cancer patients. *Journal of Psychosomatic Research;* 17: 3, 161–166

Feifel, H., Branscomb, A. (1973) Who's afraid of death? *Journal of Abnormal Psychology;* 81: 282–288.

Feigenberg, L. (1977). *Terminalvard.* Stockholm: Liber.

Feigenberg, L. (1980) *Terminal care: friendship contracts with dying cancer patients.* New York: Brunner/Mazel Publishers.

Feldstein, M., Gemma, P. (1995) Oncology nurses and chronic compounded grief. *Cancer Nursing;* 18: 3, 228–236.

Field, D. (1984) We didn't want him to die on his own: Nurses' accounts of nursing dying patients. *Journal of Advanced Nursing;* 9: 1, 59–70 .

Field, D. (1987) *Opening Up Awareness: nurses' accounts of nursing the dying.* PhD thesis. Leicester: University of Leicester.

Field, D. (1989) *Nursing the Dying.* London: Routledge/Tavistock.

Field, D., and James, V. (1993) Where and how people die. In: Clark, D. (ed). *The Future for Palliative Care: issues of policy and practice.* Buckingham/Philadelphia. Open University Press. Ch1.

Field, D. (1994) Palliative medicine and the medicalization of death. *European Journal of Cancer Care;* 3: 2, 58–62.

Field, D., Douglas, C., Jagger, C & D and, P. (1995) Terminal illness: views of patients and their lay carers. *Palliative Medicine;* 9: 45–54.

Finch, J., Wallis, L (1993) Death, inheritance and the life course. In Clark, D. (ed).*The Sociology of Death.* Oxford: Blackwell Publishers, p50–68.

Folkman S.. Lazarus, R.S. (1984) *Stress, appraisal and coping.* New York: Springer.

Forrest, D. (1989) The experience of caring. *Journal of Advanced Nursing;* 14: 815–823.

Forster, L.E., Lynn, J. (1989) The use of physiologic measures and demographic variables to predict longevity among inpatient hospice applicants. *The American Journal of Hospice Care;* March/April. 31–34.

Frankle, V. (1962) *Man's Search for Meaning.* New York: Beacon Press.

Franklin, B.L. (1974) *Patient Anxiety on Admission to Hospital.* London: Royal College of Nursing.

Freihofer, P., Felton, G. (1976) Nursing behaviours in bereavement: an exploratory study. *Nursing Research;* 25: 332–7.

Freud, S. (1957) *Thoughts for the Times on War and Death.* Standard edition: vol: XIV. London: The Hogarth Press and The Institute of Psychoanalysis.

Fulton, R. (1965) Discussion of a symposium on attitudes toward death in older persons. *Journal of Gerontology;* 16: 44–66.

Garfinkel, H. (1967) *Studies in Ethnomethodology.* Englewood Cliffs, New Jersey: Prentice Hall,

Garland, T.N., Bass, D., Otto, M.E. (1984) The needs of hospice patients and primary caregivers: a comparison of primary caregivers' and hospice nurses' perceptions. *American Journal of Hospice Care;* 1: 13, 40–45.

Gaut, D.A. (1986) Evaluating caring competencies in nursing practice. *Topics in Clinical Nursing;* 8: 2, 77–83.

References

Geissler, E. (1990) An exploratory study of selected female registered nurses: meaning and expression of nurturance. *Journal of Advanced Nursing*; 15: 5, 525–530.

Giddens, A. (1991) *Modernity and Self Identity: Self and Society in the late Modern Age.* Cambridge: Polity Press.

Glaser, B.G., Strauss, A.L. (1965) *Awareness of Dying.* New York: Aldine.

Glaser, B., Strauss, A.L. (1967) *The Discovery of Grounded Theory.* Chicago: Aldine.

Glaser, B.G., Strauss, A.L. (1968) *Time for Dying.* Chicago: Aldine.

Goffman, E. (1961) *Encounters: two studies in the sociology of interaction.* Indianapolis: Bobbs–Merrill.

Goffman, E. (1971) *The Presentation of Self in Everyday Life.* Harmondsworth: Penguin.

Goffman, E. (1983) The interaction order. *American Sociological Review.* 48: 1–17.

Gold, R.L. (1958) Roles in sociological field observations. *Social Forces*; 36: 217–223.

Gordon, R. (1978) *Dying and Creating: a search for meaning*; (Vol 4). London: Society of Analytical Psychology Ltd.

Gorer, G. (1965) *Death, Grief and Mourning.* London: Cresset Press.

Gottschlack, L.A. (1969) cited by Mostyn, B. (1985) The content analysis of qualitative research data: a dynamic approach. In: Brenner, M., Brown, J., Canter, D. (eds). *The Research Interview.* Academic Press.

Gow, K.M. (1982) *How Nurses' Emotions Affect Patient Care: self studies by nurses.* New York: Springer Publishing Company.

Gullickson, C. (1993) My death nearing its future: a Heideggerian hermeneutical analysis of the lived experience of persons with chronic illness. *Journal of Advanced Nursing*; 18: 9, 1386–1392.

Graham, H. (1983) Caring: a labour of love. In. Finch, J., Groves, D. (eds). *A Labour of Love: women, work, and caring.* London: Routledge & Kegan Paul.

Greenberg, I. (1965) *Studies of attitudes towards death: in group for advancement of psychiatry.* New York Mental Health Material Centre. Vol 5 symposium 11.

Griffin, A. (1983) A philosophical analysis of caring in nursing. *Journal of Advanced Nursing*; 8: 4, 289–295.

Hakim, C. (1987) *Research Design.* London: Allen & Unwin.

Hammersley, M. (1992) *What's Wrong with Ethnography?* London: Routledge.

Handal, P.J., Rychlak, J.F. (1971) Curvilinearity between dream content and death anxiety and the relationship of death anxiety to repression sensitization. *Journal of Abnormal Psychology*; 77: 11–16.

Hanfling, O. (1992) *Life and Meaning.* London: Blackwell Scientific Publications.

Harre, R. (1986) Is the body a thing? *International Journal of Moral and Social Studies*; 1: 3, 189–203.

Hawkins, A.H. (1991) Constructing death: three pathographies about dying. *Omega*; 22: 4, 301–317.

Heidegger, M. (1926) *Being and Time* (trans. J. Macquarrie & E. Robinson). Oxford: Blackwell.

Herth, K. (1990) Fostering hope in terminally ill people. *Journal of Advanced Nursing*; 15: 11, 1250–1259.

Hinton, J. (1963) The physical and mental distress of the dying. *Quarterly Journal of Medicine*; 32: 1–21.

Hinton, J. (1966) Facing death. *Journal of Psychosomatic Research*; 10: 22–28.

Hinton, J. (1971) Assessing the views of the dying. *Social Science and Medicine*; 5: 37–43.

Hinton, J. (1975) The influence of previous personality on reactions to having cancer. *Omega*; 6: 95 –111.

Hinton, J. (1979). Comparison of places and policies for terminal care. *The Lancet*; January 6; 1(8106): 29–32.

Hinton, J. (1984) *Dying.* Harmondsworth: Penguin.

Hoblit, P. (1972) *An Investigation of Changes in Anxiety Level following Consideration of Death in Four Groups.* Unpublished Dissertation. Baton Rouge: Louisiana State University.

Hockley J. (1989) Caring for the dying in acute hospitals. *Nursing Times;* 85: 39, 47–50.

Honeybun, J., Johnston, M., Tookman, A. (1992) The impact of a death on fellow hospice patients. *British Journal of Medical Psychology;* 65: 67–72.

Hughes, J. (1986) Denial in cancer patients. In Stoll, B.A. (ed) *Coping With Cancer Stress.* Netherlands: Martinus Nijhoff Publications, Ch7.

Hull, M.M. (1990) Sources of stress for hospice caregiving families. *The Hospice Journal:* 6: 2, 29–52.

Hull, M.M. (1991) Hospice nurses: Caring support for caregiving families. *Cancer Nursing;* 14: 2, 63–70.

Hutchinson, S.A. (1990) The case study approach. In: Moody L.E. (ed). *Advancing Nursing Science Through Research.* London: Sage Publications.

Iamarino, N.K. (1975) Relationship between death anxiety and demographic variables. *Psychological Reports;* 17: 262.

Illich, I. (1976) *Limits to Medicine.* Harmondsworth: Penguin.

Jacono, B.J. (1993) The foundational principles of leadership. *Journal of Nursing Administration;* 18: 2, 192–194.

Jackson, J. (1994) Chronic pain and the tension between the body as subject and object. In Csordas, T.J. (ed) *Embodiment and Experience: the existential ground of culture and self.* Cambridge: Cambridge University Press.

James, N. (1986) *Care and Work in Nursing the Dying: A participant study in a continuing care unit.* Phd Thesis. Aberdeen: University of Aberdeen.

James, N. (1989) Emotional labour: Skill and work in the social regulation of feeling. *Sociological Review;* 37: 1, 15–42.

James, N., Field, D. (1992) The routinisation of hospice: charisma and bureaucratisation. *Social Science and Medicine;* 34: 12, 1363–1375.

James, N. (1993) Divisions of emotional labour: disclosure and cancer. In Fineman, S. (ed) *Emotions in Organisations.* New York: Sage Publications.

James, W. (1890) *The Principles of Psychology.* New York: Holt.

Johnson J (1991) Learning to live again: adjustment following a heart attack. In Morse, J., Johnson, J. (eds) *The Illness Experience: dimensions of suffering.* New York: Sage Publications.

Jones, S.A. (1993) Personal unity in dying: Alternative conceptions of the meaning of health. *Journal of Advanced Nursing;* 18: 1, 89–94.

Jorgensen, D.L. (1989) *Participant Observation: a methodology for human studies.* London: Sage Publications.

Junker, B.H. (1960) *Field Work.* Chicago: University of Chicago Press.

Kaczorowski, J.M. (1989) Spiritual well–being and anxiety in adults diagnosed with cancer. *The Hospice Journal;* 5: 4, 105–115.

Kalish, R.A. (1979) The onset of the dying process. In Kalish, R.A. (ed) *Death, Dying, Transcending.* New York: Baywood Publishing Company.

Kastenbaum, R., Aisenberg, R. (1972) *The Psychology of Death.* New York: Springer Publishing Inc.

Kastenbaum, R. (1988) Safe death in the post–modern world. In Gilmore, A., Gilmore, S. (eds). *A Safer Death: Multidisciplinary Aspects of Terminal Care.* New York: Plenum Press.

Kastenbaum, R., Kastenbaum, B. (1989) *The Encyclopaedia of Death.* Phoenix: Oryx Press.

Kastenbaum, R., Thuell, S. (1995) Cookies baking, coffee brewing: toward a contextual theory of dying. *Omega;* 31: 3, 175–187.

Kastenbaum R. (1985) Do we die in stages? In Datan N., Ginsberg, L.H (eds). *Life Span Developmental Psychology: Normative Life Crises.* London: Academic Press.

Kayser–Jones, J., Kapp, M.B. (1989) Advocacy for the mentally impaired elderly: a case study analysis. *American Journal of Law and Medicine;* 14: 4, 353–376.

Kellehear, A. (1993). *Dying of Cancer: The final year of life.* Reading: Harwood Academic Publishers.

Kellehear, A. (1994) Are we a death denying society? A sociological review. *Social Science and Medicine;* 9: 713–723.

Kelly, M.P., May, D. (1982) Good and bad patients: a review of literature and a theoretical critique. *Journal of Advanced Nursing;* 7: 147–156.

Kiger, A.M. (1994) Student nurses' involvement with death: The image and the experience. *Journal of Advanced Nursing*; 20: 4, 679–686.

Kitson, A. (1985) On the concept of nursing care. In: Fairbairn, G. & Fairbairn, S. (eds) *Ethical Issues in Caring*. Aldershot: Avebury.

Kitson, A. (1993) *Nursing: Art and Science*. London: Chapman and Hall.

Kniesel, C. (1968) Thoughtful care of the dying. *American Journal of Nursing*; 68: 3, p550.

Krieger, S., Epsting, F., Leitner, L.M. (1974) Personal constructs, threats, and attitudes toward death. *Omega*; 5: 299.

Kübler–Ross, E. (1969) *On Death and Dying*. New York: Macmillan.

Lader, M., Marks, I. (1971) *Clinical Anxiety*. London: Heinnemann.

Lader, M.H. (1969) Psychophysiological aspects of anxiety. In Lader, M.H., (ed), *Studies of Anxiety*. Kent: Headley Bros. Ltd.

Larson, P.J. (1984) Important nurse caring behaviours perceived by patients with cancer. *Oncology Nursing Forum*; 11: 6, 46–50.

Larson, P.J. (1986) Cancer nurses' perceptions of caring. *Cancer Nursing*; 9: 2, 86–91.

Larson, P.J. (1987) Comparison of cancer patients' and profesional nurses' perceptions of important nurse caring behaviour. *Heart and Lung*; 16: 2, 187–193.

Lawler, J. (1991) *Behind the Screens: Nursing, somology and the problem of the body*. London: Churchill Livingstone.

Lazarus, R.S. (1966) *Psychological Stress and the Coping Process*. New York: McGraw–Hill.

Lee, R.M. (1993) *Doing research on sensitive topics*. London: Sage.

Leininger, M. (1986) Care facilitation and resistance factors in the culture of nursing. *Topics in Clinical Nursing*; 8: 2, 1–2.

Leininger, M.M. (1988) *Care — discovery and uses in clinical and community nursing*. Thorofare, New Jersey: Charles B. Slack.

Lester, D. (1967) Experimental and correlational studies of the fear of death. *Psychological Bulletin*; 67: 27–36.

Lester, D. (1972) Religious behaviours and attitudes towards death. In Godin, A (ed). *Death and Presence.* Brussels: Lumen Vitae Press.

Lester, D., Templer D. (1993) Death anxiety scales: a dialogue. *Omega;* 26: 4, 239–253.

Lewis, A. (1967) Problems presented by the ambiguous word 'anxiety' as used in psychopathology. *Israel Annals of Psychiatry and Related Disciplines;* 5: 105–121.

Lichter, I. (1987) *Communication in Cancer Care.* Edinburgh: Churchill Livingstone, Ch7.

Lichter, I., Hunt, E. (1990) The last 48 hours of life. *Journal of Palliative Care;* 6: 4, 7–15.

Lichter, I. (1991) Some psychological causes of distress in the terminally ill. *Palliative Medicine;* 5: 138–146.

Lieberman, M. (1965) Psychological correlates of impending death. *Journal of Gerontology;* 20: 181–190.

Lincoln, Y. S., Guba, E.G. (1985) *Naturalistic Inquiry.* London: Sage.

Lindley–Davis, B. (1991) Process of dying — defining characteristics. *Cancer Nursing;* 14: 6, 328–333.

Littlewood, J. (1992) *Aspects of Grief.* London & New York: Tavistock/Routledge.

Littlewood, J. (1993) The denial of death and rites of passage in contemporary societies. In Clark, D. (ed). *The Sociology of Death.* Oxford: Blackwell.

Llewellyn N. (1992) *The Art of Death.* London: Reaktion Books Ltd.

Lofland, J. (1971) *Analysing Social Settings.* Belmont , California: Wadsworth.

Lowry, R. (1965) *Male–Female Differences in Attitudes Towards Death.* Ph. D Thesis. Watham, Massachusetts: Brandeis University.

Lyall, W.A.L, Rogers, J., Vachon, M.L.S. (1976) *Professional stress in the care of the dying.* Palliative Care Service Report. Montreal: Royal Victoria Hospital.

Lyall, W.A.L., Vachon, M.L.S., Rogers, J (1980) A study of the degree of stress experienced by professionals caring for dying patients. In Ajemian,

I., Mount, B. (eds), *The Royal Victoria hospital Manual on Palliative/Hospice Care: a resource book.* New York: ARNO press.

Lynam, M. (1990) Examining support in context: A redefinition from the cancer patient's perspective. *Sociology of Health & Illness*; 12: 2, 169–194.

Maguire, P. (1985) Barriers to psychological care of the dying. *British Medical Journal*; 291: December 14; 291 (6510): 1711–3.

Mant, A. K. (1968) The medical definition of death. In Toynbee, A., Mant, K., Smart, N., Hinton, J., et al (eds). *Man's Concern with Death.* Hodder & Stoughton.

Marks–Maran, D. (1992) Rethinking the nursing process. In Jolley, M., Brykczynska, G, (eds), *Nursing Care: The challenge to change.* London: Edward Arnold.

Martinson, I., Neelon, V. (1995) Physiological characteristics of dying and death. In Corless I.B., Germino, B., Pittman, M. (eds) *Dying, Death and Bereavement.* London: Jones & Bartlett Publishers.

Mayer, D.K. (1986) Cancer patients' and families' perceptions of nurse caring behaviours. *Topics in Clinical Nursing*; 8: 2, 63–69.

Mayeroff, M. (1971) *On Caring.* New York: Harper & Row.

McCarthy, J. (1980) *Death Anxiety.* New York: Gardner Press Inc.

McFarlane, J. (1988) Nursing: a paradigm of caring. In: Fairbairn, G., Fairbairn, S. (eds) *Ethical Issues in Caring.* Aldershot: Avebury.

McGinnis, S.S. (1986) How can nurses improve the quality of life of the hospice client and family? An exploratory study. *The Hospice Journal*; 2: 1, 23–36.

McLean, G. L. (1993) *Facing death: conversations with cancer patients.* London: Churchill Livingstone.

McMahon, R., Pearson, A. (1992) *Nursing as a Therapy.* London: Chapman and Hall.

Mead, G.H. (1934) *Mind, Self and Society.* Chicago: University of Chicago Press.

Mead, G.H. (1964). In: Strauss, A. (ed) *On Social Psychology: Selected papers.* Chicago: University of Chicago Press.

Meier, P., Pugh, E.J. (1986) The case study: a viable approach to clinical research. *Research in Nursing and Health*; 9: 3, 195–202.

Melia, K. (1987) *Learning and Working: The occupational socialization of nurses.* London: Tavistock Publications.

Mellor, P.A., Shilling, C. (1993) Modernity, self identity and the sequestration of death. *Sociology*; 27: 3, 411–431.

Menzies, I. (1960) *A Case Study in the Functioning of Social Systems as a Defence against Anxiety.* London: Tavistock.

Merleau–Ponty, M. (1962) *The Phenomenology of Perception.* London: Routledge and Kegan Paul.

Meyer, J.E. (1975) *Death and Neurosis.* New York: International Universities Press.

Miles, M.B., Huberman, A.M. (1994) *Qualitative Data Analysis.* London: Sage Publications.

Mitchell, Clyde, J. (1983) Case and situational analysis. *The Sociological Review*; 3: 187–211.

Morrison, P. (1991) The caring attitude in nursing practice: a repertory grid study of trained nurses perceptions. *Nurse Education Today*; 11: 1, 3–11.

Morse, J., Solberg, S., Neander, W., Bottorff, J., et al (1990) Concepts of caring and caring as a concept. *Advances in Nursing Science*; 13: 1, 1–14.

Morse, J. (1991) Negotiating commitment and involvement in the nurse–patient relationship. *Journal of Advanced Nursing*; 16: 4, 455–468.

Morse, J.M, Bottorff, J., Anderson, G., O'Brien, B., et al (1992) Beyond empathy: expanding expressions of caring. *Journal of Advanced Nursing*; 17: 7, 809–821.

Mostyn, B. (1985) The content analysis of qualitative research data: a dynamic approach. In: Brenner, M., Brown, J., Canter, D. (eds). *The Research Interview.* London: Academic Press.

Mount, B., Cohen, R., MacDonald, N., Bruera, E. et al (1995) Ethical issues in palliative care research revisited. *Palliative Medicine*; 9: 2, 165–170.

Muetzel, P. (1988) Therapeutic nursing. In: Pearson, A. (ed). *Primary Nursing; nursing in the Burford and and Oxford Nursing Development Units.* London: Croom Helm.

References

Mulkay, M., Ernst, J. (1991) The changing profile of social death. *European Journal of Sociology*; 32: 172–196.

Munhall, P. (1988) Ethical considerations in qualitative research. *Western Journal of Nursing Research*; 10: 2, 150–162.

Nagy, M. (1959). The child's view of death. In: Feifel, H. (ed), *The Meaning of Death..* New York: McGraw–Hill.

Newbury, A (1991) The care of the patient near the end of life. In: Penson, J., Fisher, R. (eds). *Palliative Care for People with Cancer.* London: Edward Arnold.

Norton, J. (1963) Treatment of a dying patient. *Psychoanalytic Study of the Child;* 18: 541–560.

Nuland, S. (1994) *How We Die: reflections on life's final chapter.* New York: A.A. Knopf.

Obbens, E. (1993) Neurological problems in palliative medicine. In: Doyle, D., Hanks, G.W.C. & MacDonald, N. (eds). *Oxford Textbook of Palliative Medicine;* Oxford: Oxford Unversity Press.

Osler, W. (1906) *Science and Immortality.* London: Constable.

Parkes, C.M., Weiss, R.S. (1983) *Recovery from Bereavement.* New York: Basic Books.

Parkes, C.M., Parkes, J. (1984) Hospice versus hospital care: re–evaluation after ten years as seen by surviving spouses. *Postgraduate Medical Journal;* 60: 120–124.

Pattison, E.M. (1977) *The Experience of Dying.* New Jersey: Prentice–Hall Englewood–Cliffs.

Pearsall, M. (1965) Participant observation as role and method in behavioral research. *Nursing Research;* 14: 37–42.

Pearson, P. (1991) Clients' perceptions: The use of case studies in developing theory. *Journal of Advanced Nursing;* 16: 5, 521–528.

Peterson, S., Greil, A. (1990) Death experience and religion. *Omega;* 21: 1, 75–82.

Phillips, D. F. (1972) The hospital and the dying patient. *Hospital;* 46: 4, 68.

Pine, V.R. (1980) Social organization and death. In: Kalish, R. A. (ed) *Death, Dying, Transcending.* New York: Baywood Publishing Company Inc.

Quint, J.C. (1967) *The Nurse and the Dying Patient.* New York: Macmillan.

Qvarnstrom, U. (1978) *Patients' Reactions to Impending Death.* Stockholm: Institute of International Education & Department of Medicine.

Ragin, C.C., Becker, H.S. (1992) *What is a case? Exploring the foundations of social inquiry.* New York: Cambridge University Press.

Rainey, L. (1988) The experience of dying. In: Wass, H., Berardo, F., Neimeyer, R. (eds) *Dying: Facing the facts.* 2nd edn. Washington: Hemisphere.

Ramos, M.C. (1992) The nurse–patient relationship: theme and variations. *Journal of Advanced Nursing;* 17: 4, 496–506.

Rando, T.A. (1984) *Grief, Dying and Death.* Illinois: Research Press Company.

Rando, T.A. (1988) Anticipatory Grief: The term is a misnomer but the phenomenon exists. *Journal of Palliative Care;* 4: 1, 70–73.

Rasmussen, B., Norberg, A., Sandman, P. (1995) Stories about becoming a hospice nurse: reasons, expectations, hopes and concerns. *Cancer Nursing;* 18: 5, 344–354.

Ray, M.A. (1981) A philosophical analysis of caring within nursing. In: Leininger, M (ed) *Caring: An essential human need. Proceedings of three national caring conferences.* Thorofare, New Jersey; Charles Slack.

Reimer J.C., Davies, B., Martens, N. (1991) Palliative care: the nurse's role in helping families through the transition of 'fading away'. *Cancer Nursing;* 14: 6, 321–327.

Reuben, D.B, Mor, V. Hiris, J. (1988) Clinical symptoms and length of survival in patients with terminal cancer. *Archives of Internal Medicine;* 148: 1586.

Robson, C. (1993) *Real World Research.* Oxford: Blackwell Publishers.

Rosenthal, M.A., Gebski, V.J., Kefford, R.F., Stuart–Harris, R.C. (1993) Prediction of life expectancy in hospice patients: identification of novel prognostic factors. *Palliative Medicine;* 7: 199–204.

Russell, G.C. (1993) The role of denial in clinical practice. *Journal of Advanced Nursing;* 18: 6, 938–940.

Ryan, P.Y. (1992) Perceptions of the most helpful nursing behaviours in a home–care hospice setting: Caregivers and nurses. *American Journal of Hospice & Palliative Care;* 9: 5, 22–31.

Samarel, N. (1991) *Caring for Life and Death.* London: Hemisphere Publications.

Sartre, J.P. (1958) *Being and Nothingness.* (trans. H.E. Barnes). London: Metheun.

Saunders, C. (1959) *Care of the Dying.* London: Macmillan.

Saunders, C. (1970) Care of the dying. *Nursing Times;* 72: 26, 3–24.

Saunders, C., Summers, D., Teller, N. (1981). *Hospice — the Living Idea.* London: Edward Arnold.

Saunders, C. M. (1985) *The Management of Terminal Illness.* 2nd ed. London: Edward Arnold.

Saunders, C. (1989) Pain and impending death. In: Wall, P. D., Melzack, R. (eds). *Textbook of Pain.* 2nd edn. Edinburgh: Churchill Livingstone.

Schulz, R. (1978) Death Anxiety: Intuitive and empirical perspectives. In: Bugen, L.A. (ed) *Death and Dying: Theory, research, practice.* Iowa: W.C. Brown Company Publishers.

Schulz, R., Alderman, D. (1974). Clinical research and the stages of dying. *Omega;* 5: 137–143.

Schou, K.C. (1990) Awareness contexts and the construction of dying in the cancer treatment setting: Micro and macro levels in narrative analysis. In: *The Sociology of Death.* (Clark, D., ed). Oxford: Blackwell Publishers.

Seale, C. (1989) What happens in hospices: a review of research evidence. *Social Science Medicine;* 28: 6, .551–559.

Seeland, I. (1991). The process of dying. In: Seeland I., Klagsbrun, S., DeBellis, R., Kutscher, A., Avellanet, C., Dennis, J. (eds). *The Final 48 Hours.* Philadelphia: The Charles Press Publishers.

Shalom, A. (1989) *The Body/mind Conceptual Framework and the Problem of Personal Identity.* Atlantic Highlands, New Jersey: Humanities Press International.

Shearer, R.E. (1973) Religious Beliefs and Attitudes towards Death. *Dissertation Abstracts International;* 33: 3292–3293.

Simpson M.A. (1979) *Dying, Death and Grief: a critically annotated bibliography and source book of thanatology and terminal care.* New York: Plenum Press.

Skorupha, P., Bohnet, N. (1982) Primary caregivers perceptions of nursing behaviours that best meet their needs in a home care hospice setting. *Cancer Nursing;* 5: 5, 371–374.

Smart, N. (1968a) Philosophical concepts of death. In: Toynbee, A. Mant, K., Smart, N., Hinton, J., et al (eds). *Man's Concern with Death.* London: Hodder & Stoughton.

Smart, N. (1968b) Some inadequacies of recent Christian thought about death. In: Toynbee, A., Mant, K., Smart, N., Hinton, J., et al (eds) *Man's Concern with Death.* London: Hodder & Stoughton.

Smith, D. C. (1993) The terminally ill patient's right to be in denial. *Omega;* 27: 2, 115–121.

Smith, M.J. (1990) Caring: Ubiquitous or unique. *Nursing Science Quarterly;* 3: 2, 54.

Smith, N. (1990) The impact of terminal illness on the family. *Palliative Medicine;* 4: 127–135.

Smith, P. (1988) *Quality of Nursing and the Ward as a Learning Environment for Student Nurses: A multimethod approach.* PhD Thesis. London: Kings College, University of London.

Smith, P. (1992) *The Emotional Labour of Nursing.* London: Macmillan Education.

Speilberger, C.D. (1966) *Theory and research on anxiety.* In: Speilberger, C.D. (ed) *Anxiety and Behaviour.* New York: Academic Press.

Standing Medical Advisory and Standing Nursing and Midwifey Advisory Committee Joint Working Party on Palliative Care (1992). *The Principles and Provision of Palliative Care.* Department of Health: London.

Stedeford, A. (1988) *Facing Death: Patients, families and professionals.* London: Heinemann.

Stockwell, F. (1972) *The Unpopular Patient.* London: Royal College of Nursing Publications.

Stone, G.P. (1962) Appearance and the Self. In: Rose, A. (ed) *Human Behaviour and Social Processes.* Boston: Houghton Mifflin.

Strauss, A. (1959) *Mirrors and Masks*. New York: Free Press.

Strauss, A., and Glaser, B. (1970) *Anguish — a case history of a dying trajectory*. California: The Sociology Press.

Strauss, A., Corbin, J. (1990) *Basics of Qualitative Research: grounded theory procedures and techniques*. London: Sage Publications.

Stroebe, M.S. (1992) Coping with bereavement: A review of the grief work hypothesis. *Omega*; 26: 1, 19–42.

Stroebe, M.S., Stroebe, W., Hansson, R.O. (1993) *Handbook of bereavement: Theory, Research and Intervention*. New York: Cambridge University Press.

Sudnow, D. (1967) *Passing On: The social organization of dying*. Eaglewood Cliffs, New Jersey: Prentice–Hall.

Sweeting, H.N., Gilhooly, M.L. (1992) Doctor, am I dead? A review of social death in modern societies. *Omega*; 24: 4, 251–269.

Taylor, H. (1983) *The Hospice Movement in Britain: its role and its functions*. London: Centre for Policy on Aging.

Taylor, S.E. (1983) Adjustment to threatening events. *American Psychologist*; (November) 38: 1161–1173.

Templer, D. (1970) The construction and validation of a death anxiety scale. *Journal of General Psychology*; 82: 165–177.

Templer, D., Ruff, C., Franks, C. (1971) Death anxiety: Age, sex, and parental resemblance in diverse populations. *Developmental Psychology*; 4: 108.

Templer, D. (1972) Death anxiety in religiously very involved persons. *Psychological Reports*; 31: 361–362.

Templer, D. (1976) Two factor theory of death anxiety. *Essence*; 2: 91–94.

Tolor, A., Reznikoff, M. (1967) Relationship between insight, repression–sensitization, internal–external control, and death anxiety. *Journal of Abnormal Psychology*; 72: 426–430.

Tolstoy, L. (1960) *The Death of Ivan Ilyich and Other Stories*. Harmondsworth: Penguin.

Toynbee, A. (1968) Changing attitudes towards death in the modern western world. In: Toynbee, A., Mant, K., Smart, N., Hinton, J., et al (eds). *Man's Concern with Death*. Hodder & Stoughton.

Toynbee, A., Mant, K., Smart, N., Hinton, J., et al (1968) *Man's Concern with Death*. London: Hodder & Stoughton.

Tross, S., Holland, J. (1989) Psychological sequelae in cancer survivors. In: Holland, J., Rowland, J. (eds). *Handbook of Psychooncology: Psychological care of the patient with cancer*. Oxford: Oxford University Press.

Turner, B.S. (1984) *The Body and Society: Explorations in social theory*. Oxford: Blackwell.

Twycross, R.G., Lichter, I. (1993) The terminal phase. In: Doyle, D., Hanks, G.W.C., MacDonald, N. (eds) *Oxford Textbook of Palliative Medicine*. Oxford: Oxford Medical Publications.

Vachon, M.L.S. (1986) Myths and realities in palliative/hospice care. *The Hospice Journal*; 2: 1, 63–80.

Vachon, M.L.S. (1978) Motivation and stress experienced by staff working with the terminally ill. *Death Education*; 2: 113– 22.

Vachon, M.L.S., Lyall, W.A. L., Freeman, S.J.J. (1978) Measurement and management of stress in health professionals working with advanced cancer patients. *Death Education*; 1: 365–375.

Vachon (1993) Emotional problems in palliative medicine; patient, family and the professional. In: Doyle, D., Hanks, G.W.C., MacDonald, N. (eds), *Oxford Textbook of Palliative Medicine*. Oxford: Oxford Medical Publications.

Van Gennep, A. (1960) *The Rites of Passage*. Chicago: University of Chicago Press.

Veatch, R.M. (1989) *Death, Dying and the Biological Revolution*. New Haven & London: Yale University Press.

Ventafridda, V., Ripamonti, C., de Conno, F., Tamburini, M., et al (1990) Symptom prevalence and control during cancer patients last days of life. *Journal of Palliative Care*; 6: 7–11.

Walter, T. (1991) Modern death: Taboo or not taboo? *Sociology*; 25: 2, 293–310.

Walter, T. (1994) *The Revival of Death*. London & New York: Routledge.

Watson, J. (1985) *Nursing: The Philosophy and Science of Caring*. Boston: Little, Brown & Co.

Weisman, A.D. (1972) *On Dying and Denying: A psychiatric study of terminality*. New York: Behavioural Publications Inc.

References

Weisman, A.D. (1979) *Coping with Cancer.* New York: McGraw–Hill.

Weisman, A.D. (1984) *The Coping Capacity: On the nature of being mortal.* New York: Human Sciences Press Inc.

Weisman, A., Hackett, T. (1967) Denial as a social act. In: Levin, S., Kahana, R., (eds) *Psychodynamic Studies on Aging: Creativity, reminiscing and dying.* New York: International Universities Press.

Weisman, A.D. (1992) Commentary on Corr's 'A task–based approach to coping with dying.' *Omega;* 24: 2, 95–96.

Weisman, A.D., Kastenbaum, R. (1968) *The Psychological Autopsy. A study of the terminal phase of life.* New York: Behavioural Publications.

Weisman A.D. (1974) *The realisation of death. A guide for psychological autopsy.* New York: Jason Aronson.

Weisman A.D. (1988) Appropriate death and the hospice program. *The Hospice Program;* 4: 1, 65–76.

Wilkes, E. (1980) *Report of the Working Group on Terminal Care.* London: DHSS.

Wilkinson, S. (1991) Factors which influence how nurses communicate with cancer patients. *Journal of Advanced Nursing;* 16: 6, 677–688.

Wilson–Barnett, J., Richardson, A (1993) Nursing research and palliative care. In: Doyle, D, Hanks, G.W.C., MacDonald, N. (eds) *Oxford Textbook of Palliative Medicine;* Oxford: Oxford Medical Publications.

Witzel, L. (1975) Behaviour of the dying patient. *British Medical Journal;* 2: 81–82.

Wolf, Z.R. (1986) The caring concept and nurse identified caring behaviours. *Topics in Clinical Nursing;* 8: 2, 84–93.

Worden, J.W. (1991) *Grief Counselling and Grief Therapy.* 2nd ed. London: Routledge.

World Health Organization (1990). *Cancer Pain Relief and Palliative Care: Report of a WHO Expert Committee.* Geneva: WHO Technical Report Series.

Wright, K., Dyke, S (1984) Expressed concerns of adult cancer patients' family members. *Cancer Nursing;* 7: 5, 371–374.

Yin, R. (1989) *Case Study Research: design and methods.* London: Sage.

Zlatin, D,M. (1995) Life themes: a method to understand terminal illness. *Omega;* 31: 3, 189–206.

Znanieki, F (1934) *The Method of Sociology.* New York: Farrar & Rinehart.

Index

acceptance 13, 14, 37, 38, 39, 202
act of closure 31
act of holding on 157, 193
act of letting go 157, 193
act of not talking openly 114
act of pacing 122
act of protecting 110
  protecting kin 110, 133
  protecting nurse 110, 119
  protecting patients 119, 133
  protecting self 110, 123, 124,
  125, 128, 133
act of talking openly 111
act of waiting 155
act of watching 155
acting as a go-between 116, 117,
  119, 133
acts of
  controlling 199, 210
  holding on 199, 210
  letting go 199, 210
  protecting 199, 210
  watching and waiting 199, 210
acts of holding on
  and letting go 68
acts of protecting
  and controlling 68
acts of watching and waiting 68
acute crisis phase 43, 44
after-life 6, 167
age, sex, marital status 229
agitation 10
analysis and interpretation
  of data 57
  macro-level of analysis 57

analytical versus statistical
  generalisation 221
anger 37, 44, 48, 89, 94, 149
anticipated loss 5
anticipatory grief 5, 206, 207
anxiety 7, 12, 16, 33, 72, 91
anxiousness 85
attachments of the
  present life 171, 200
awareness of dying 40
  closed awareness 40, 41
  mutual pretence
  awareness 40, 41
  open awareness 40, 41
  suspicion awareness 40, 41
awareness of dying and
  impending death vii

bargaining 37, 44
bereaved 5, 45, 206
bodily deterioration 135
body 48, 171, 172
body-person split 158, 171, 172,
  174, 193, 208, 210
breaking the connection 32
breathlessness 10, 72, 73, 85, 86,
  98, 180, 201

cancer survivors 82, 202
care work 27, 200
caring for dying people 25
case histories 53
case studies 53, 54, 219, 220, 221,
  222, 223, 229, 230
categories 51, 62, 67, 68
  main core category 63
  sub-categories 63
childhood developmental
  theory 38
Christianity 5, 6, 62, 81, 88, 93, 99,
  102, 167, 169
chronic living-dying phase 43

closed awareness   48
closure   200, 243
coding   60, 68, 69, 109, 219
coding paradigm   61, 67
collective dying   205
comparative analysis   63
conceptual mapping   67, 68, 209
confusion   11
consciousness   11
constructs of caring   27
context of awareness theory   40
control over others   110
coping mechanisms   13, 23
coping with dying   14, 46
counsellor   240
cremation   66, 84, 104, 116, 172
critical juncture   59, 174, 198
cross-case comparisons   59, 67, 109
cross-checking   69
curative treatment   v

day centre   77, 75, 81, 84, 88, 91,
   96, 99, 100, 103, 108, 204, 226,
   227, 228
death anxiety and age   16
death anxiety and ill health   17
Death Anxiety Scale   16
death management   200
death preferences   162
death saturation   30
death-anxiety   52
defence behaviours   33
defence mechanisms   12, 33, 43
Definitions of death   4
demographic data   57, 230
denial   12, 13, 14, 37, 44, 48, 157,
   177, 202, 203, 216
First-order denial   14
frank and partial denials   14
Second-order denial   14
Third-order denial   14

dependence   170, 199
depression   17, 37
dread   7, 12
duration   134
dying role   82, 143, 146
dying trajectories   41, 42, 49, 82,
   109, 110, 134, 143, 157, 174, 202,
   207, 208, 224, 229
dying trajectory
   duration   49
   form   49
   individual's   42
   shape   49
dying/non-dying role   202
dyspnoea   10, 11, 184, 185

ego function   13
embarrassment   21, 122, 123,
   149, 199
embodiment of self   209
emotional aspects   200, 201
emotional involvement   29, 30
emotional labour   27
empowerment   46, 48, 199
epicureanism   5
Epiphanic experiences
ethical considerations   224
ethical issues   6
ethnographic   51
euthanasia   78, 159, 160
everyday-life activities   110
existentialism   5, 6

face-to-face relationships   219
family life-cycle   16, 22, 201, 206,
   208
family systems theory   23
fatigue and weakness   201
fear   33, 73, 205
   death fears: 7
   of the dead
fieldwork   51, 225

five-stage model of dying 37, 39, 203
form 155
funeral 84
funeral preparations 76, 84, 172, 178

generation of categories 62, 63
good death 4, 34
grounded theory 51, 52
guidance 199

home 204
home care 152, 204, 227, 228
hospice 27, 33, 70, 71, 73, 74, 75, 81, 82, 83, 87, 93, 99, 102, 104, 106, 107, 113, 114, 127, 128, 131, 152, 155, 163, 204, 205, 206, 207, 208, 216, 217, 225, 226, 227, 228, 229, 230
hospice movement v, 217
hospice nurses 29, 34
hospice nursing 33, 202, 208
human life cycle 15

immortality 7
impending death vi, ix, 39, 199
inability to speak 181
inability to swallow 10
incontinence 10, 79, 98, 101, 104, 122, 159, 180, 201
independence 170, 199
institutionalised death 19, 20, 24, 216
integrated and disintegrated dying 44, 48
interactionism ix
   interpretive ix
   symbolic viii
interactionist framework 219
interpersonal relationships 14

interpretive interactionist framework viii
interviews with dying individuals 50, 233, 236
   funnel approach 235
involvement of nurses 29

limitations and criticisms of the study 210
lingering death 10, 24
living-dying interval 44, 45, 218
living-dying interval/phase theory of dying 43
living-dying intervals 49
long-term remission 135, 202, 210
loss of speech 201
losses 6, 45, 88, 89, 122, 128, 134, 155, 199, 206, 240, 243

macro-level of analysis 59
managing rejection 131
markers 155, 242
mature ego-coping mechanisms 15
medicalisation of death 19
mental anguish. 73
methods 54
micro-level of analysis 58, 59
middle knowledge 14
mind and body 208
model death 162, 163, 164, 166
morbid fears 4
mortality rates 20
mosaic 39, 155
multi-dimensional aspects of dying 49, 201
multiple methodological approaches 220
mutual pretence 48
nausea 134, 147
nausea and vomiting 10, 11, 12, 78, 85, 91, 94, 97, 103

noisy breathing   10, 73
not open about dying   114
numerous deaths   34
nurse-patient encounters   28, 110, 123, 158, 211, 219
nurse-patient relationship   vi, 27, 28, 29, 35,198, 199, 201, 215, 239
nurses and caring   24, 25
nursing behaviours   31
nursing education   198, 207, 208
nursing practice   207

observer-as-participant   232
ontological security   18
open about dying   111
open awareness   48, 203, 216, 217, 218

pain   7, 10, 11, 26, 33, 34, 70, 73, 77, 78, 79, 81, 93, 94, 95, 96, 99, 104, 105, 119, 134, 137, 138, 147, 153, 180, 188, 189, 191, 201, 209
palliative care   v, vii, 26, 83, 88, 91, 93, 98, 99, 140, 225
participant observation   51, 211, 212, 221, 232
participant-as-observer   232
past my sell-by date   109, 134, 139, 142, 148, 155
paternalism   224
patient-nurse encounters   199, 200, 219
patient-nurse/nurse-patient encounter   70
patient-on-nurse watching   155
patient-on-patient watching   135, 155
patient-on-self watching   135, 155
patient/nurse relationship   198, 199

patients' dignity   242
patterns of dying   63, 175, 176, 210
    person not ready, body not ready   191, 210
    person not ready, body ready   182, 210
    person ready, body not ready   176, 210
    person ready, body ready   179, 210
peaceful death   193, 208
performance status   11
personal control   110
personal fading   135, 147, 154, 155
personal identity   ix, 219
personal support   240
physical decline   182
physical deterioration   10, 45, 120, 134, 136, 138, 139, 147, 154, 158, 163, 171, 193, 201, 204, 206, 207, 216, 236
physical fading   135, 147, 155
plateau   44, 88, 107
population   221
preparation for death   47
preparations for one's funeral   125
presentation of self   132, 219
principal tools   54
private front   120, 132
probability sampling   222
problematic situations   198, 205
process of dying   4, 8, 18, 197, 205
prospective studies   216
protecting kin   69
protecting nurse   69
protecting self   69
protracted dying   159, 161
psychoanalysts   7
psychoanalytical approaches   12
psychodynamic orientation   12
psychological adjustment   202

psychological autopsy 52
psychological tests 52
public and private fronts 121, 124, 132
public front 120, 157

questionnaires 52

readiness to die 209
readiness to die 156, 174, 175, 179, 193, 208, 210
redefining self 123, 197, 198, 203
reliability of data 211
religion and death anxiety 16, 17
researcher effect 211, 212
respect 199
restlessness 10, 11
rituals 18, 19, 20
Rorschach inkblot test 52

sampling 221, 222
self and the body 18, 171, 172, 208
self-protection 133
sensitive topics 224
separation 8, 209
sequential aspects of dying 49
social death 21
social fading 135, 147, 152, 155
social influences 18, 19, 203
socially alive 204
socially dead 204
somological nursing 122, 209
spiritual dimensions 38, 173
stage theory of dying 36, 37, 38, 40, 203
stigma 82
stoicism 5
struggle 165, 193, 205, 207
survival 192, 202
surviving 194
suspended-sentence trajectory 143

suspicion awareness 48
symbolic-interactionist approach 51
symbolic-interactionist perspective viii, 219
symptoms (and life expectancy) 11
synchrony of dying 174
systematic comparisons 51
systems theory 22

taboo 3
taking each day as it comes 110, 133, 134
taking risks 199
task work 46
task-based approach to coping with dying 45, 47
terminal phase 43, 44, 47, 109, 143, 157, 193
the process of dying
living with the process of dying 9
themes 51
theories on death and dying 36, 210
theory of the body 209
third-order denial 203
three-stage model of dying 39
transcript of recorded interview 59
transitions 23, 210
treatment calendar 22, 110
treatment regimes 81
treatments 87, 88, 139, 141, 156, 183, 189, 193
truth-telling culture 48
turning-point experiences

unconsciousness 162
unexpected death 35
unidimensional approach 40, 49

urinary dysfunction   10
use of interpretative methods   211

validity of the data   211
vital processes   12
vomiting   134, 147
vulnerable groups   224

weak   94, 108
weakness   93, 204